SPECIAL PRAISE FOR

weightless

"Only Gregg could tell a story that's this dark with this much humor. He brings hope to the most desperate situations in a refreshing and inspiring way."

—REGINA KING
ACTOR/DIRECTOR/PRODUCER

"In 2005, after winning NBC's *The Biggest Loser*, I thought I had it all figured out. I was thin, had some extra jingle in my pocket, and had met the woman who would later become my wife. I was so confident that I was on the right track with my weight and the struggles I had overcome, I even wrote a book to tell others how they could be just like me. The weight stayed off for a while, but it steadily came back, pound by single pound.

"As I regained weight, the problem wasn't that I didn't know what to do, rather it was the fact that I was so embarrassed and ashamed. Not only did I struggle with feeling like a failure, but also with an unhealthy body image. Guys aren't supposed to worry about body image, right?

"Years after being celebrated around the world for my transformation, I was at a pretty low point when I was asked to read Gregg McBride's book, *Weightless*. It could not have come at a better time. Gregg's story demonstrates that regardless of circumstances, we all have the power to change and maintain a healthy weight. He helps us understand that often, it isn't the weight at all that is holding us back. The thing that holds us back is our own minds.

"As someone who has struggled mightily with my weight and feeling 'not good enough,' I can proudly say that this book has helped me to find my way again. I'm sure it will do the same for you!"

—MATT HOOVER
WINNER, *THE BIGGEST LOSER* (SEASON 2)

"*Weightless* is a delicious read in every way. In this funny, wise, and emotionally honest book, Gregg McBride offers hope and inspiration to weight-challenged people longing for change and acceptance without sacrificing their true selves."

—CATHERINE WHITNEY
COAUTHOR, *EAT RIGHT 4 YOUR TYPE*

"*Weightless* takes your heart to the gym and gives it a real workout. Gregg McBride's struggle with weight reminds us how important the emotional connection with food really is. His ability to have you smiling (and crying) through it all speaks volumes about his strength. As someone who reads a lot of weight loss books, I'm a fan."

—LORI CORBIN
FOOD AND FITNESS COACH, KABC-TV LOS ANGELES

"Gregg's journey is refreshing and compelling because he gets to the heart of what it *really* takes to get rid of excess weight. He deftly addresses the mental and physical work necessary to lose weight and keep it off for good."

—DIANE CARBONELL
AUTHOR, *150 POUNDS GONE FOREVER*

"This isn't your typical before-and-after story. In these exceedingly candid, poignant, and at times downright hilarious pages, Gregg probes the tragic past that fueled his broken relationship with food, and reveals the physical, emotional, and psychological metamorphosis that accompanied his 250-plus-pound weight loss. Tracing his journey up and down the scale, Gregg shares how he finally broke free from the dangerous 'on-off' diet mentality, and how you can, too."

—JOHANNAH SAKIMURA, MS
EVERYDAY HEALTH NUTRITION BLOGGER

"*Weightless* is an astonishingly honest, hilarious, heartbreaking, and uplifting story of physical, emotional, and spiritual transformation. It is easy to imagine Gregg's story ending tragically if not for his indomitable spirit, his infectious humor, and his many creative talents. *Weightless* is an inspiring read, even if you've never been a pound overweight."

—FRANCESCA HOGI
SURVIVOR: REDEMPTION ISLAND
SURVIVOR: CARAMOAN
MATCHMAKER

weightless

GREGG
MCBRIDE

weightless

*My Life as a Fat Man
and How I Escaped*

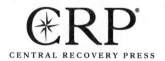

CENTRAL RECOVERY PRESS

LAS VEGAS

Central Recovery Press (CRP) is committed to publishing exceptional materials addressing addiction treatment, recovery, and behavioral healthcare topics, including original and quality books, audio/visual communications, and web-based new media. Through a diverse selection of titles, we seek to contribute a broad range of unique resources for professionals, recovering individuals and their families, and the general public.

For more information, visit www.centralrecoverypress.com.

Publisher: Central Recovery Press
3321 N. Buffalo Drive
Las Vegas, NV 89129

19 18 17 16 15 14   1 2 3 4 5

ISBN: 978-1-937612-69-6 (paper)
978-1-937612-70-2 (e-book)

Publisher's Note: This is a memoir, a work based on fact recorded to the best of the author's memory. Central Recovery Press books represent the experiences and opinions of their authors only. Every effort has been made to ensure that events, institutions, and statistics presented in our books as facts are accurate and up-to-date. To protect their privacy, the names of some of the people and institutions in this book have been changed.

The advice contained herein is intended as a reference only, not as a medical manual. The information given here is designed to help you make informed decisions about your health. It is not intended as a substitute for any treatment that may have been prescribed by your doctor. If you suspect you have a medical condition, you are urged to seek competent medical help. A qualified medical professional should always be consulted for his or her approval before beginning any new diet or any other health or exercise program. The author and the publisher expressly disclaim responsibility for any adverse effects arising from the use or application of the information contained herein.

The recipes contained in this book should be followed exactly as written. The author and the publisher expressly disclaim responsibility for your specific health or allergy needs that may require medical supervision. The author and the publisher expressly disclaim responsibility for any adverse reactions to the recipes contained herein.

Also, mention of specific companies, organizations, or authorities does not imply endorsement by the author or publisher, nor does mention of specific companies, organizations, or authorities imply that they endorse this book.

Some of the information in this book has been previously published by the author. Excerpts from his book, *Just Stop Eating So Much!* (Bridesmade, Inc., 2007) and his blog juststopeatingsomuch.com are used with permission.

Photos used are from author's personal collection.
Author photo by Robin Ganter Photography. Used with permission.

Cover design and interior design and layout by Marisa Jackson

For anyone carrying the
burden of excess weight—
whether mental or physical—
this one's for you.

table of contents

foreword

Gregg came into my life in a most unexpected way, through an email snafu of all things. Looking back, this was rather appropriate given his penchant for originality and razor-sharp wit. Gregg is someone you can't meet without coming away smiling—if not laughing out loud. Thus, I'm grateful for the unexpected.

In my many years of meeting Joy Fit Club members who lost 100 or more pounds simply by relying on diet and exercise, I remember being awestruck by Gregg's back story. Here was someone who took off over 250 pounds and kept it off for over a decade, despite living through so many years of sadness and abuse. I found it hard to connect the man with such a sad past I was reading about with the one I was emailing—the fun, happy, and joke-filled person who clearly has a real appetite for life.

Upon meeting Gregg in person at his first *Today* show appearance, my crush was in full swing. Not only was he game for wrapping hosts Kathie Lee Gifford and Hoda Kotb in his sixty-inch belt—something the ladies didn't know about until we were on the air—but he asked if he could enter the studio as if he were on a Paris catwalk and then complain that he thought he was there for a segment on modeling. Needless to say, his on-air spot was a smashing success and the entire studio was laughing on volume *ten*.

This is the kind of spirit and—well, *joy*—that gets me excited as well as inspired. I know Gregg has been motivating others for years with his blog and the projects he writes for film and television. Even if he's creating a new horror-themed project for Hollywood, you can find moments of whimsy and relief in his work. I think it's these kinds of moments that have the potential to touch all of our lives in positive ways.

When Gregg told me about this book, I actually beat him to the punch and asked if I might be able to write the Foreword. (He said he was going to ask me, but who knows if that's true?)

I'm glad I'm the one doing it, because I find Gregg's story so compelling and uplifting. On the one hand, because of the honesty with which he looks back at the horrific experiences in his past that shaped the reasons he over-ate to the point of weighing over 450 pounds. On the other hand because, at the same time, he finds his own responsibility to himself and to his mental and physical health in a truly refreshing way.

Gregg has always been a writer (and, perhaps, a ham) at heart, which means he's kept track of things in a way that many others who've won the battle of the bulge have not. He is able to detail the family and social adversities he faced, as well as many of the actual binges he partook in to prevent himself from being all that he had the potential to be. And, oh, what a potential that is.

That same potential is available to all of us, no matter how many times we've tried to succeed in the past. This time can be different. It was for Gregg. It can be for you. Personally, I can't help but be motivated every time I re-familiarize myself with Gregg's story.

The honest kind of perspective offered in this book is what makes Gregg who he is today, and I've seen the impact people are left with—no matter if they're trying to lose weight or face another life-changing challenge—when they hear his personal story.

I'm excited Gregg finally committed this story to publication so that it can be shared with the many others who also have the power to overcome anything they're facing or, as Gregg puts it, who have the power to become *weightless*.

—Joy Bauer, MS, RD, CDN
Nutrition and Health Expert for NBC's *Today* Show
New York Times best-selling author of
Joy Bauer's Food Cures and *Your Inner Skinny*
Contributing Editor/Monthly Columnist to *Woman's Day*

acknowledgments

Honestly, I'm not sure who I'd like to thank more—the people in my life who have provided me with the most encouragement or those who've provided me with the most challenge. Both have given me so much. I'm truly grateful. And to those whom I've challenged over the years (and the list is lengthy)—whether or not we are still a part of one another's lives, please know that when I think of you, it's with respect, appreciation, and admiration.

This book, which chronicles said challenges (and triumphs) has been a longtime dream of mine. It never would have come to fruition without the encouragement and inspiration from the esteemed Joy Bauer, Amy Goldsmith, and Catherine Whitney, as well as my brilliant attorney Kim Stenton, my dedicated (and über-hot) screenwriting agents Debbie Deuble-Hill and Sheryl Petersen, and my book agents Steve Fisher and the ultra-dedicated Linda Konner—each of whom has been with me throughout every step of this journey.

Similarly, the entire team at Central Recovery Press (Patrick Hughes, Valerie Killeen, and my amazingly talented editors, Eliza

Tutellier and Nancy Schenck) has shared their talents, guidance, and support wholeheartedly (and not just because they wanted me to continually email them pictures of my dog—although I'm sure that perk didn't hurt). And to graphic designer Marisa Jackson, I am grateful for the meaningful and iconic book cover (and interior) design. Your talents shine!

There are others who have been instrumental to this specific work as well—including the fifteen gifted friends and family members who made direct contributions through their write-ups included herein. This book would not be what it is without your wonderful insights and reflections. Joy, your Foreword and friendship both mean the world to me. And Petra, your Thin/Fat Observations that you've graciously allowed me to share on these pages continually bring me clarity, determination, and laughter. Hear that applause? That's from me, to you. And Jaxon, your allowing me to feature your beautiful song lyrics is a gift I carry with me every day. You, my friend, are a true hero.

I'd also like to thank the people who remind me daily that "family" comes in all sorts of incarnations. To Charlene, Elizabeth, Grace, Kath, Maggie, Michele, Nik, Peter, Sally, Yvonne, and Jason, I thank you from the bottom of my heart for loving and accepting all aspects of who I am. You lift me on a daily basis and I am forever grateful. And to Latte, my seven-pound bundle of fur, who continually teaches me that there's bliss in every moment, I am eternally grateful for the reminders and all of the smooches.

Lastly, I'd like to thank you, the reader. And this is not done in an effort to encourage you to keep reading. The journey I share is one of highs, lows, and lots of in-betweens. Having you on this path with me, even simply via these pages, helps my strength and my resolve, which can in turn hopefully help and inspire yours.

We're all in this together. And for that, I sincerely thank you.

the weight-ing game

I am standing in darkness, having been hidden away by my host.

I'm not sure what's happening at this moment or why I was shoved into this dark room and told not to touch anything or make any sounds.

I can hear people passing by in the hallway. Who are these people? Why am I not allowed to see them? Are they embarrassed of me? Have I done something wrong?

I am overcome with paranoia and anxiousness—feelings I'm all too familiar with after everything I've experienced in my life. The abuse from my parents that I thought was normal and sometimes felt was deserved, getting teased and tortured throughout my school days (even into college), not fitting in (often literally) wherever I went, and, saddest of all, not believing in myself enough to not let any of these things matter.

Is the event that I'm here for—something I thought was going to be so wonderful—to be another letdown? Am I here to fall flat on my face? Is this going to be my destiny forever? To continue to fail?

As I begin to wipe sweat from my brow, the door opens. I hold my breath.

Light streams into the room and I am yanked out into the hallway and shoved toward a doorway.

"When that door opens, walk through it," says the gruff voice of the man who's shoving me forward. I turn to get a closer look at him but he disappears just as quickly as he appeared, having entered a side office.

I am once again alone.

My heart is pounding. I try to breathe, but my chest is tightening up.

"This was a mistake," I tell myself. "I never should have accepted this invitation. But it's too late now. I've got to go through with it."

I look toward the doorway I was instructed to walk through. I realize this is it. This is going to be, like it or not, a defining moment.

Am I going to sink or swim?

I summon up the courage to do everything it takes to soar, as the door in front of me begins to open. As I step forward I can't make out anything but bright lights. I'm squinting to see what's waiting for me on the other side. But I'm blinded by the lights.

I realize what's about to happen is going to change everything.

gregg's weight by book section

PART I	
AGE	WEIGHT
Birth	8 lbs. 6 oz.
8	175 lbs.
12	225 lbs.
14	275 lbs.
17	300 lbs.
18	325 lbs.

PART II	
AGE	WEIGHT
18	325/335 lbs.
20	400 lbs.
22	464 lbs.
23	457.5 lbs.
27	450 lbs.
28	435 lbs.
29	185 lbs.
30	285 lbs.
30	185 lbs.

PART III	
AGE	WEIGHT
31	175 lbs.
Today	175 lbs.
I no longer weigh myself regularly!	

A G E	W E I G H T
Birth	8 lbs. 6 oz.
8	175 lbs.
12	225 lbs.
14	275 lbs.
17	300 lbs.
18	325 lbs.

PART I

before

growing pains

God got it wrong.

In his infinite wisdom he created magnificent mountains, shimmering oceans, and Sandra Bullock's smile. But when it came to food groups, he screwed up big time. I mean, why can't carrots be high in fat and chocolate be good for your eyes? What was the Almighty thinking? Then again, what was *I* thinking?

At six years old, I was a scrawny, skinny little kid. All I would eat was hot dogs and oatmeal—and not necessarily on the same day. I have vague memories of being coerced into eating more by my parents who were worried about their growing boy. Needless to say, I taught them a thing or two about growing.

My father was an officer in the Air Force, so we moved around a lot. I was born in Germany, then we moved to Indiana, where my sister Lori was born, and later to Tennessee. After Tennessee we moved to Hanscom Air Force Base in Bedford, Massachusetts, where we stayed for a number of years while the military sent my dad to Harvard to earn his MBA.

As a child, a lot of my eating habits were self-taught. In fact, once I started gaining weight, I was forbidden from having any snacks or sweets. Because I wasn't allowed to have "junk food," I was drawn to it in every eating situation that occurred when my parents weren't around. I would use my allowance to buy contraband candy, and that became my addiction—my drug of choice, if you will. All because I never learned moderation.

By the time I turned eight, I was indulging in cheating cycles. Anytime I purchased snacks or junk food with my allowance, I knew I had to eat it by the time my parents got home. At age six, I couldn't drink a whole can of Coke, but by age eight I could down eight Mr. Goodbars in one sitting. I didn't know it at the time, but I was already cultivating the fine art of bingeing.

Eight-Year-Old Gregg's Typical Binge

8-pack of Mr. Goodbar Chocolate Bars

1 Charleston Chew Candy Bar

2 cans of Pepsi

As the years went on, so did the weight (well, it *added* on, anyway).

I remember in third grade, I was actually the center of a mini-gambling syndicate due to my size. My classmates were making bets based on how heavy they thought I was. And at the time, I couldn't have been prouder. I was amused by it all and, being a wannabe celebrity, or at least a wannabe popular kid, I was beginning to embrace any form of attention, no matter how negative the spotlight may have been.

I waited happily until all the bets were placed, there was usually a lunchtime deadline, and then stepped on a scale outside of the gym during lunch hour. I had to weigh before I ate my lunch—that was the rule. The smart set began to bet that I'd always be heavier. And they were right. I was soon weighing in at over 175 pounds.

My mom was in the hospital off and on during this period due to complications from what we were told was multiple sclerosis, putting my father in charge of cooking. He used to serve me cottage cheese, lettuce, and a burger patty—the "official back-in-the-day diet meal." After dinner, I would retreat to my bedroom and indulge in my secret stash of cookies and candy. I would also buy gallons of ice cream and keep it hidden in my closet until I could eat it. Needless to say I would more often end up drinking rather than eating it.

With my mom in the hospital, my dad seemed to be suffering from a lot of anxiety, which is perhaps what led to his increased drinking, often at all times of the day. Fitness is a big deal for the military-minded, and the last thing my dad wanted was an overweight son. But the more he pushed for me to get thin, the more I ballooned. His rules got more and more rigid, to the point where I wasn't able to have any food from the bread group. This included rice, potatoes, and anything else of a starchy nature.

One late afternoon, before my father got home from work, I pulled out a box of "forbidden" saltine crackers and some cheese slices. After putting mayonnaise on the crackers I placed a piece of cheese on top, followed by a pickle slice. I guess I always was a junior Emeril Lagasse at heart! I laid all of my hors d'oeuvres out on a plate and prepared to take it to my bedroom, the safe haven for my undercover munching.

Suddenly—*tap-tap-tap*. I looked up at the window (we lived in a basement apartment) and saw my dad banging on the window, smiling sarcastically, proud to have caught me "cheating" on my diet. He came inside and made me sit at the kitchen table to watch him enjoy the snack I had worked so hard to create.

"I'm not going to punish you," he said. "Instead, I'm going to thank you for fixing me such a delicious snack."

That's okay though. Because, boy, did I show him.

The next morning, while my dad was in the shower, I took a ten-dollar bill from his wallet and spent it all on candy after school. Back then ten dollars actually bought quite a bit of snack food. After coming home, I went deep into the woods behind our building and proceeded to force the entire contents of the bag of junk into my belly. I was so sick when I finished eating that I felt like throwing up. I didn't know much about supermodels or eating disorders at that time, so I didn't realize throwing up on purpose might have been an option. An unhealthy option, but an option nonetheless.

While I learned to hide what I was eating, I was having more and more trouble hiding its effect on my body. My parents now had to order my clothes from the Sears big and tall catalog, and once, at a grade school birthday party, I was eating a slice of birthday cake when the wicker chair I was sitting on buckled and collapsed.

The other kids laughed, while the kid's mom who was hosting the event launched into a lecture on how I was eating too much cake. I don't remember any specific parts of her lecture. As she pointed her finger and ranted, I ground my tongue into the roof of my mouth, still able to decipher the granules of sugar that had been in the frosting. Sugar saved me from feeling completely mortified.

I realize now that was about the moment I began to hate my body. It seemed like the bigger I got, the more my parents (and others) became comfortable with letting me know that I was not only differently, but also incorrectly sized. It wasn't difficult to see the disgust in other peoples' faces or the disappointment in my parents' eyes. I seemed to be failing everyone. And it was apparently my growing belly's fault. So I reasoned, if they hated my body, why shouldn't I?

I remember one time, after getting yelled at by my mother for eating some of her candy (which she kept hidden in her bedroom and I was forbidden to touch); my father confessed that he was the one who had eaten it. While my mom and dad stood in the kitchen, debating whether or not I should still be punished, since in their eyes I must have been guilty of sneaking some kind of food since I was continuing to gain weight, I remember listening to them while coloring in the living room. I began to write "I am bad. My parents are good. I hate myself" in the coloring book. It was soon after that "incident" that I started to keep a private journal, knowing I couldn't risk my newly discovered self-hating thoughts getting into my sister's (or worse yet my parents') hands.

While I occasionally made a spectacle of myself when encountering wicker furniture and was now battling a case of chronic self-loathing, I was still fairly popular at school. By the fifth grade, I had assumed the position of class clown, always a fitting complement to excess poundage. While kids were busy making money from my ongoing weight gains, I was also charging kids ten cents each to watch me kiss my "girlfriend," Ann, behind the big rocks that sat at the base of our grade school.

Can you guess where my earnings were going?

Unfortunately, Ann's and my passion for each other was fleeting. Our love affair ended not because I wasn't Catholic, the reason fifth-grade Ann gave me as to why we could never marry, but because people began to make fun of Ann for kissing the fat kid. Our breakup was a terribly sad experience. Luckily, Little Debbie and her cavalcade of snack cakes saw me through that painful period.

Learning to "eat my problems away" was a pervasive habit I developed early in life. If I had any cause to be anxious, depressed, or worried, I'd head to the store and spend ten dollars on ice cream, cookies, chips—you name it.

Just around the time I learned that I could "eat away" my depression, I was faced with more things to feel depressed about. My father's alcoholism was becoming a noticeable issue, and it was escalating. He was facing legal action from the Air Force for one-too-many DUIs. Meanwhile, my mother, who had been recuperating from years in the hospital due to complications from her MS, saw fit to forget her worries by having an affair.

My younger sister Lori, who happened to be thin and beautiful, and I had a succession of baby-sitters who were around more often than our parents. I remember one in particular, Sue, who would let me sit next to her while she watched television. I was actually allowed to snuggle up to her, something I was never encouraged to do with my parents. I felt Sue's warmth and affection, and most importantly, her acceptance. I was further delighted by Sue's obsession with dunking potato chips in mustard. I thought it was genius.

Pairing two unrelated snack foods together? Sign me up.

Some of my happiest childhood memories are of dunking potato chips with Sue.

The baby-sitter situation turned ugly when my parents hired George, a seventeen-year-old, who sexually abused me. After the first incident George said that if I told anyone he would kill me—a threat that seemed very real at the time. He showed me his pocketknife to prove the point. I believed him. And I was terrified.

When my parents arrived home that evening, I got up out of bed and went into their bedroom where my mother was taking off her make-up. I told her I needed to talk, and she told me that if I didn't get back to bed I was going to get a spanking. I tried to reason with her but she wasn't responsive at all—and clearly was very serious about the spanking. I went back to my room and cried myself to sleep.

George continued abusing me whenever he would baby-sit. My parents didn't understand why I would get "testy" whenever it was announced that he would be watching us. I kept a drawer full of candy bars at the ready on nights when I had advanced warning of George's visits. During his abuse, I would detach from what was happening and think only of the food that would comfort me when the ordeal was over.

Eventually George went off to college and I was safe from his abuse at last. But by that point I had formed an unbreakable bond with food, and food promised to "be there" for me and to protect me from any of life's future unbearable situations.

This was about the time my parents decided that they wished they had never met one another—much less had children together. My sister Lori and I had a sense that our presence was bothersome. The situation was made worse when we moved to North Andover, Massachusetts, where we had to make new friends in the middle of a school year, a time when most school friendships are already cemented.

To Lori's and my credit, we began to counter the negative feelings at home by excelling in theater programs at school. Lori had the advantage of being thin and beautiful, assuring her of leading roles. My weight kept me relegated to the "ha-ha" character roles or in the last row of the chorus. But that was good enough for me. Even without any lines to speak, I could still be someone else on stage. Not being me for an hour or two felt like an enormous relief.

When my mom and dad did direct their attention toward me, they were on me to lose weight. One day they'd yell at me, the next they would try and bribe me with the promise of some new gadget just to "encourage" me to lose weight. None of it worked. For in the world of junk food, I was safe, warm, and loved. No one could harm me while I was eating candy and chips, no matter how sick I felt after eating too much of them.

There were some surprising benefits to bingeing. When all I could think of was how sick, bloated, and close to "exploding" I felt, I wouldn't have to think of anything else. I didn't have to think about being ignored by my parents, or about being molested by the baby-sitter, or about the fact that most kids at school wouldn't look in my direction, much less talk to me. I'd discovered a safe, if physically painful, haven where not even my thoughts, memories, or fears could do me any harm.

I continued taking money from my dad's wallet to fund my ever-growing junk-food habit. He must have been confused about what amount he'd spent at bars the previous night to notice that money was missing. And that was fine by me.

By sixth grade, I was spending roughly ten dollars a day on junk food, which bought quite a bit on a military base since food prices are discounted for service people and their families. I would turn down offers to go play with my few friends after school so I could buy junk food instead and go home and eat it in front of the television.

Sixth-Grade Gregg's Typical Binge

1 "party size" bag of Hershey Miniature Candy Bars

1 large bag of Lays Potato Chips

1 bottle of Barbecue Sauce (for "dip")

1 can of Whipped Cream

1 gallon of Neapolitan Ice Cream

6-pack of Fanta Orange Flavored Soda

My fondest memories of being in sixth grade are when I pretended to be sick and stayed home from school. I would be home alone since both my parents worked, so I would go to the store to buy a ton of junk food and then watch *Brady Bunch* reruns during the noon hour.

Oh, what joy I experienced—until the day when my dad came home midday and caught me sitting up, eating nine different things and watching TV. Being sick in our home meant you were supposed to stay in bed all day without any television.

Dad asked me for an explanation. I said I had just woken up and that the TV was already on and that it was somebody else's food on the coffee table.

Dad stared at me for about a half a minute and then proclaimed, "Somebody must be setting you up." He told me to go back to bed and never mentioned the incident again. He did confiscate my stash of junk food, however. But no matter, one quick trip to his wallet the next morning and I was able to replenish my supplies.

My "chronic sickness" bit me in the butt when my parents finally consulted a doctor, who checked me into the hospital for two days to undergo a series of tests, determined to find out what was wrong. I was terrified the tests wouldn't find anything physically wrong with me, but I have happy memories of being in the hospital for those two days. It was Easter weekend and candy stripers kept dropping by with candy and cookies. Even in the hospital my binge behavior worsened; just ask the sick kid I shared my room with who had his Easter basket ransacked, while he was sleeping, by the "sick" kid lying in the bed next to him.

The tests didn't reveal any hidden sickness, but they did confirm a severe dust allergy. I was relieved the doctor's found "something," so I wasn't exposed as the kid who was just constantly playing hooky.

FOREIGN AFFAIRS

By seventh grade, we went to live in Singapore for a year. Having clothes tailor-made there was cheaper than buying off the rack, and as a result I don't think anyone in my family noticed that I kept getting bigger and bigger. There were no bothersome size labels to document my progress.

My father's drinking continued to escalate, as did my mother's affairs. I was only eleven years old at that point and didn't yet have the mental capacity to understand the reasons for all the angst in our home, but things were getting so dysfunctional that in between eating and bingeing, I would often attempt to run away from home.

The problem with running away from home in Singapore is that the island is only twenty-six miles wide and sits in the middle of the Indian Ocean.

Where did I think I was going?

I would take a bus to the edge of the island, get scared, and then take a cab back home. Of course I didn't have money for the taxi, so I'd have to go into the house and ask my parents for the cab fare. Then I'd get in trouble not only for running away, but also for needing the cab money.

I ran away from home more than seven different times over the course of the year we lived in Singapore. One night I tried scaling down the side of our house from the second floor. Needless to say my 225-pound girth kept me from being successful. I got stuck on a window ledge and had to call for help until my parents finally heard me and grudgingly came to my rescue.

Seventh-Grade Gregg's Typical Binge

4 Hot-Dogs-with-Everything at the local A&W

2 large orders of Onion Rings

1 large A&W Root Beer

1 Chocolate Milk Shake

1 Vanilla Milk Shake

My favorite friend in Singapore also happened to be named Sue. She was our full-time housekeeper—a luxury far more affordable in Singapore—and boy, oh boy, could she cook. What's more, she was delighted to see me enjoy food as much as I did, and she was always willing to fix me something to eat. Food equaled love. And I wanted all the "love" I could get.

My father's drinking continued to affect his career in the Air Force, and it wasn't long before we were transferred again—this time to Landstuhl, Germany. This was about the time all hell broke loose at home.

My father was on TDY, meaning "Temporary Duty Yonder," the military's slang for a business trip, which kept him away from home most of the time.

Meanwhile, my mother was plotting to become the most desired "natural" blonde in our small military community. We were sternly instructed to say that blond was my mother's real hair color even though we knew it came from a box. She was working for the public affairs office at Landstuhl Hospital, where she became the belle of the ball. Men, both single and married, began calling the apartment in droves. It was at this time that my mom hatched what she thought was an ingenious plan for me to screen her calls.

Mom insisted that whenever the phone rang, no one was to answer it but me, and that I was to assume the identity of Sue, our *female* maid in Singapore, who still lived there and had not traveled with us to Germany. My still-high-pitched voice and tendency toward theatrics fit into her plan very nicely. Being twelve, I had no real understanding of what I was doing.

So I would answer the phone, pretending to be Sue, the female maid, and basically handled my mother's dating schedule. It got to a point where various men would call "Sue," i.e., me, for advice on how to win my mother's affection. And when my mom would blow them off, they even started asking "Sue" out on dates.

I thought I was handling this insanity perfectly fine. I enjoyed the thrill of performing and, more importantly, I had my secret world of food ever at my disposal. Now I also had the "bonus" of my mom's approval and perceived affection for doing her bidding. Little did I realize at that point my mom could have given a Disney-inspired villain a run for his or her money when it came to cruel ways to parent a child.

Since Mom was always away from home on dates, including overnight stays and long weekends, I was able to maintain a nice stash of junk food. It began to extend beyond sweets and candy. Whenever I could, I would fix whole meals for myself—no matter what time of day. My typical breakfast during those years was really more like lunch or dinner.

Eighth-Grade Gregg's Typical Breakfast

1 large box of Spaghetti
1 large jar of Spaghetti Sauce
1 whole can of Parmesan Cheese
1 loaf of White Bread
Butter and Garlic for the Bread

At twelve years old I was running the household—cleaning, fixing dinner, making sure that Lori and I got to school on time and that we stayed out of my mom's hair, all while coordinating my mom's social life over the telephone by pretending to be "Sue." I was writing notes to teachers and signing school permission slips by forging my mother's signature when necessary. I was a one-stop-shop, and Lori and I were a good team.

My favorite memories from that period were of Saturday mornings during the winter. My mom would usually leave around 4:00 a.m. to go skiing with the man-of-the-moment. Lori and I would pretend to be asleep until she left and then we would get up immediately afterward.

I'd race to the kitchen and fix us a big pot of spaghetti complete with tomato sauce and Parmesan cheese. It would be about 5:00 a.m. at that point. Lori and I then sat down with a tape recorder and a nearby stereo system and made an audiotape of our own version of a television variety show—ingeniously titled *The Gregg and Lori Show*. We had lots of special guests (whatever cassette tapes we had of our favorite performers) and would insert canned "applause" into our recording to make it sound like our "musical guests" were performing live.

During our recording sessions we would chow down on the spaghetti. I always ate much more than Lori, who continued to maintain a healthy weight, while my own weight continued to skyrocket.

Ramstein Junior High School, where I commuted to via bus from Landstuhl, was an interesting place. A school full of military brats (a common nickname for the kids of military personnel), each of whom was convinced that his or her father outranked all the others'.

I didn't have any close friends, so when I discovered that a kid at school named Mike shared my love of superhero comic books I used some of my precious food money to buy a few comics for him in the hopes it might bring us closer together. It worked, and before too long I had a new "best friend"—though Mike never used that exact phrase. I had never really had a good friend before, not to mention a thin friend. In some weird way, I felt a little more validated as a person.

Look, world. Someone likes me even though I'm fat!

Mike and I used to sit around and quiz each other about science fiction television episodes and comic books. We were happening guys.

Adding to this newfound social life? *Girlfriends.* One for Mike and one for me. Suddenly I wasn't solely focused on food anymore and it felt fantastic. My girlfriend's name was Judy. She had blond hair and a wicked sense of humor. Mike and his girlfriend, Kim, and Judy and I would French kiss like there was no tomorrow.

While I could tell Judy liked me, I never forgot the fact that I was fat and she was not. I was obsessed with finding out why she would have a "fat guy" as a boyfriend. Mike agreed to do the detective work for me.

One day after lunch I was waiting in the school hallway to go into class when Mike approached me with the news. Apparently Judy wanted to date me because since I was the fattest guy in school, I "probably had the biggest dick."

Never mind the compliment of my perceived appendage—my growing belly had kept me from seeing my penis when looking down for years. I was mortified at being singled out as the "fattest guy at school." I waited outside Judy's fifth period class to quiz her on these events. And she confessed. She had indeed said that.

I felt compelled to break up with Judy. Not so much because of the fat remark, but because I was somewhat disgusted by her candor. I wasn't ready to move that fast. Especially as I watched my mother demonstrate the ills of illicit sex by staying away from home night after night and gaining a public reputation for being a "slut." This word was used by more than one caller giving "Sue" a piece of his mind in regard to my mother blowing them off.

Soon after my breakup with Judy I also "broke up" with Mike. He said his mother had accused me of buying his friendship by constantly purchasing comic books for him. I told him that wasn't the case at all, and subsequently stopped buying him comics. Funny enough, he stopped being my friend about the same time he stopped getting my comic books. Go figure.

INWARD BOUND

I had a journalism teacher who caught on to something not being quite "right" with me. She assumed the problems were occurring inside me, rather than stemming from my home situation. She signed me up for the school-sponsored Outward Bound program, where I was forced to experience nature with a group of other "troubled" kids.

In actuality only a few of the kids were genuinely "troubled." Most of us were simply adjusting to adolescence in one random way or another while living on a military base overseas. We were the European equivalent of *Gossip Girl*—without the cocktails—even though, ironically, all of us could buy beer off the military base at a

German bar or pub. Its availability meant few of us military brats ever abused alcohol—and besides, I was too busy abusing food.

The Outward Bound trip proved a good way for me to get to know a few people in school. When Mike and I stopped being friends, I became very shy and withdrew into myself.

Interacting with people this closely was a new experience for me. I remember our first morning there, where five of us were assigned to the same room. There was a fellow eighth-grader, Glenn, who I became fascinated with. This was before I realized he was one of the most popular kids in school.

What fascinated me most was when Glenn was changing his shirt. The fascination wasn't sexual. His athletic body intrigued me because it was so unlike my own. Unlike my puffy, curvy, Pillsbury Doughboy body, Glenn was totally fit. He had a tight chest, so different from my growing "breasts," and he had a taut stomach. Not me. I had a huge stomach and flabby body. Even my penis, the one Judy had been so interested in, was receding into itself due to my belly's full roundness.

Seeing Glenn up close like that, I began to hate my body even more than I had before. Standing in front of the mirror, I grabbed chunks of my blubbery flesh, wondering why I couldn't look more like Glenn. I chronicled all of this in my journal—describing how my body was so much different from Glenn's.

There was hell to pay for those journal entries. On the bus ride home from the Outward Bound week, some of the kids managed to get their hands on my journal and began reading it out loud to everyone on the bus. Every last detail of my comparing my flabby body to Glenn's fit body was recounted for a bunch of eleven- and twelve-year-olds. I tried to get the teacher's attention but she wouldn't intervene. You can imagine the razzing I got. I was mortified. After that incident I held my head very low while walking the halls of Ramstein Junior High School.

Post humiliation, I showed that journalism teacher a thing or two about how "troubled" I was. I volunteered to sell yearbooks at lunch, and I was a hell of a salesman. The only caveat? I was stealing about twenty to thirty dollars a day from the profits in order to fund my food stash. My ten-dollar supply was no longer enough to satisfy me despite feeling that I was going to "explode" almost daily. I needed more money for more food. And since my parents were rarely around, I no longer had their purse or wallet as an ATM-like resource.

Each day at school, after I'd "sold" yearbooks and kept most of the profits for myself, I would run to the nearest food market during lunch, store the bags of food in my locker, then tote the groceries with me on the bus ride home. Once I got home to our apartment, I would fix whatever concoctions I wanted to create for my palate. I was now eating huge amounts on a daily basis.

Gregg's Typical Yearbook-Funded Binge

1 gallon of Chocolate Ice Cream
*(which I would wrap in foil to keep cold and less messy
since it had to be stored in my locker until I went home)*

1 jar of "Hot" Fudge Sauce

1 can of Whipped Cream

Bananas

2 large bags of Barbecue Potato Chips

1 large pack of Nutter Butter Peanut Butter Sandwich Cookies

1 large pack of Oreo Cookies

Eventually the journalism teacher tried to get to the bottom of who was stealing money from the yearbook fund. Based on how often I volunteered to man the yearbook sales table she suspected it was me, but she couldn't prove it. So she gathered the class together to talk

about shame, deceit, and how awful a person must be to sink so low, all the while visually indicating in my direction.

Then she left the room, leaving the class in charge of deciding who stole the money and to determine the thief's punishment. With all my practice of being "Sue," I was able to act innocent and, despite accusations, I never buckled under pressure. I don't think anyone really bought my act, but there was no way of proving that I had been the one stealing the money. After all, I had eaten the evidence.

In the meantime, my mother found "true love" with an army man named Keith, and he was up for meeting Lori and me. Keith decided he wanted to spend the evening at our apartment, cooking dinner for the three of us.

Dinner? That made him A-okay in my book.

The night Keith came over Mom had to work late and "Sue" had the night off. So he prepared dinner and then we waited with him in the living room. Keith quizzed Lori and me about our backgrounds. We told him all about Massachusetts, Singapore, and basically our whole life story. We loved to talk about ourselves. After all, we were the hosts and stars of *The Gregg and Lori Show* and had the cassette tapes to prove it.

To our surprise, Keith suddenly lost his appetite, told us to give his apologies to our mom, and left abruptly. When Mom came home she asked us to recount the details of the evening and then she hit the roof. She was furious that Lori and I had shared our "life history" with someone we were meeting for the first time. It turns out she had spun a web of lies for Keith. Among them, that my father didn't exist and that Lori and I were adopted.

My mother forced me to call Keith and say that Lori and I had made up all those stories about our childhood because we were ashamed of being adopted. I had to tell Keith that I had a chronic problem with lying. Finally, I was instructed to beg that he not hold our lying against our mom and ask him to forgive my sister and me. He wouldn't.

Neither would my mother. *Ever.* As I would soon learn.

Safely back in my bedroom, I proceeded to eat a bar of chocolate as tears streaked down my face. I told myself it couldn't get any worse than this.

I was wrong.

ANOTHER PERSPECTIVE
ON GREGG AT THIS TIME

By Lori McBride, Gregg's Sister

It was surprising for me, when I read these pages, to discover that Gregg felt insecure about his weight when we were children. I was younger, so maybe I wasn't always aware of the nature or the extent of the elementary school taunting, but he always seemed "larger than life" to me. No pun intended . . . really. It was as though his resiliency made him that much more determined to be noticed for something other than his weight.

Growing up in the military we moved a lot and it was thanks to Gregg's outgoing personality that we made new friends quickly wherever we moved. He always took charge in a creative way—if you wanted to have fun, you wanted to be with Gregg. He was always making a way of escape, whether by producing elaborate home movie "blockbusters," or fabricating tiny items to stock the shelves of a Barbie store, or by "producing" *The Gregg & Lori Show*. He was so quirky and original. From my viewpoint, looking up to my big brother, it seemed like everyone wanted to be his friend.

Living in Singapore as children was amazing. I remember Gregg getting a lot of attention wherever we went. The combination of his red hair, freckles, and excess weight was unusual to see in that Asian culture. He often wore football-style T-shirts that had a large number on the front and back, which seemed to bridge any language gap. Whenever we were in town, people would call out whatever number happened to be on his shirt as a way to get his attention . . . or to ridicule him . . . I guess we'll never know.

I was aware of some of Gregg's bingeing. Occasionally I was included—if only to buy my silence on the matter. One time, I remember Gregg eating ice cream in his bedroom, having emptied the carton into a Tupperware bowl. Our mom knocked on the door, so he hurriedly stashed the bowl on the floor of his closet. When he opened the door, our Irish setter, Mac, bounded in, and his nose quickly found that bowl. He began crazily lapping up the ice cream, so Mom investigated . . . and Gregg was busted.

Our parents' well-intentioned efforts to control the binge eating only served to light the fire under it. They installed locks on our kitchen cabinets and routinely inspected the garbage cans. If any contraband wrappers or containers were discovered, they were kept until weekend afternoons, when we were whipped with a belt for each offense. The ensuing misery required more binges to help him forget.

Some of the details of our upbringing are pretty hard to re-live. Through the years, it seems Gregg and I have honored an unwritten pact, as fellow survivors. The pain of our childhood can't be taken off like a coat, but must be shed more like skin . . . cell by cell.

CHAPTER TWO

foxy for a fat kid

Moving to a new town and new school right before the fourth quarter of eighth grade was no picnic. Although it did offer some relief, considering that Ramstein Junior High considered me to be a petty thief, with perhaps the biggest penis, thanks to Judy's ruminations. I had stopped stealing money for food at that point, but I never managed to regain my honor before leaving town.

Our new hometown of Wiesbaden, Germany, offered a brand new world, but one that wasn't too receptive given how late in the school year it was. After an uncomfortable quarter in junior high, I finished the year without making any new friends in the area.

Lori and I continued to lead an active fantasy life at home—constantly singing and acting into the tape recorder—ready for discovery by Hollywood at any moment. We were too clueless to realize there weren't a lot of Hollywood talent scouts in Wiesbaden, Germany.

During the summer before high school, I volunteered for the Red Cross where I met two of my soon-to-be good friends, Diana and Rhodonna. It was our shared love of *Charlie's Angels* reruns that brought us together. We spent the summer bringing playing cards to hospital patients and practicing our dancing when no one else was around.

I was volunteering at the same hospital where my mom had gotten a job, but for some reason she did not want me visiting her office. So I would call her from time to time from within the same building. Oddly, her receptionist used to correct me when I would ask for "Diana McBride." She'd say, "You mean Dee-ana." Looking back now, I realize that at that point my mom's metamorphosis into the blonde vixen of the Wiesbaden Military Hospital was already under way. But back then, I just thought the receptionist was being passive aggressive.

As my dad was no longer on TDY (away on business), the plan was for him to live with us at the apartment.

One big happy family. *Not*.

Dad was still drinking heavily and would come home late at night from his alcohol binges at the Officer's Club. He'd wake up early in the morning and leave for work and return very late at night. We barely saw him.

My mother used this time to paint a terrible picture of how "bad" my dad was. One morning I woke up to her telling me that my dad had completely disgusted her. Delighted to have my mother confide in me and seeing it as a potential bonding experience, I asked her what was wrong. She told me she had gotten up in the middle of the night and had found my dad in the kitchen, masturbating while looking at the bra section of the Sears catalog.

Why my mother, *any* mother, would tell an impressionable adolescent boy this story—about his own father, no less—is beyond me. It skewed my view of masturbation and sex for years to come.

Soon after that my father moved out and lived away from home—though we were not allowed to admit that to anyone. If we did, we'd risk losing the military housing we were living in, since the service person in question wasn't actually living there. Lori and I were instructed to act like we were the normal military family, which, ironically, we were—marital strife is quite rampant among military families.

So Lori and I pretended Dad still lived with us for the sake of our military-sanctioned housing. While I no longer had to be "Sue," I was still the appointment secretary for my mom and dad. Eventually my mom instructed me to answer the phone with "Diana McBride's residence." And so I did. Every time the phone rang, I'd answer "Diana McBride's residence."

I was never as good at saying "Dee-ana" as my mom's receptionist at the hospital. Perhaps that's why Mom would acknowledge the receptionist's presence in public, but would barely acknowledge mine.

Dad came around once a week, usually on Saturday mornings. He would pick up the grocery list and go shopping. I was responsible for compiling the list. Needless to say I couldn't request any type of sweets or junk food—in fact, I was supposed to be on a strict diet assigned, via a badly Xeroxed handout, from a doctor at the hospital.

The diet's day plan was a joke. That a doctor would put a growing teenage boy on a diet like that is a testament to what the medical community did not know about dieting or healthy eating at the time.

High School Gregg's Joke of a Diet: Typical Day

BREAKFAST

2 pieces of Wheat Toast

Pat of Butter

½ Grapefruit

LUNCH

½ cup Cottage Cheese

Lettuce Leaves

1 sliced Tomato

1 Fruit of Choice

AFTERNOON SNACK

No afternoon snack, you're fat!

DINNER

½ cup Tuna Fish

1 tbsp. Mayonnaise

Lettuce Leaves

Canned Vegetables of Choice

1 Fruit of Choice

EVENING SNACK

½ cup Bouillon

I developed my own interpretation of the diet.

High School Gregg's Joke of a Diet: Typical Day (Gregg's Variation)

BREAKFAST

2 pieces of Wheat Toast

Pat of Butter

½ Grapefruit

LUNCH

½ cup Cottage Cheese

Lettuce Leaves

1 sliced Tomato

Fruit of Choice

1 can Fresca Diet Soda

AFTERNOON SNACK

1 large bag of Potato Chips

2 Hot Dogs

2 to 4 Candy Bars (any variety)

DINNER

1 can of Zucchini in Tomato Sauce

1 can of Tuna Fish

1 large package of Cheddar Cheese, melted

1 can Fresca Diet Soda

EVENING SNACK

1 gallon of Chocolate Ice Cream

1 bag of Oreo Cookies

(Mixed together—way before "Cookies and Cream"
was a thing—someone stole my original idea!)

6 cans of Fresca Diet Soda

The diet "additions" I would procure myself. My dad would only buy food at the market that he deemed "healthy or diet-approved." Dad's weekly shopping routine was always a drag.

After he brought the groceries home, we would gather in the living room as a family. This was when my mother would present my father with a list of what I had done wrong the previous week. Dad would then take off his belt. I would have to drop my pants and underwear. And then my mom would watch as my dad spanked me for a week's worth of bad deeds.

It was horrible and I would always end up crying. I'm not sure which was worse—the physical pain or the mental anguish. One time I was crying so loudly that Mom told my dad to stop. For a moment I thought she was rescuing me from his forceful blows. Instead she said, "Hold on a minute. We don't want the neighbors hearing him cry." They waited for me to calm down and then resumed the spanking.

Lori didn't suffer this wrath as often as I did. I was doing my best to form a protective layer around her. And for some reason, my parents seemed to respect that. It was as if anything my mom or dad had to say to Lori would be disseminated through me. I was basically in charge of raising both Lori and myself. Dad wasn't there except for Saturdays, and Mom was never around, except when she brought stray men to the apartment for torrid sex sessions.

From time to time Lori and I did have major arguments. I was always "on" her to get dressed or to do her homework. I was the "parent" in charge of making lunches, cooking dinner, and doing everything else in between. But even during the arguments, Lori and I always remained a team—along with our Irish setter, Mac, who loved us both dearly.

All this time Mom and Dad continued harping about my weight. Cheating on my diet was worthy of a spanking or two on Saturday afternoons. My father took me to the hospital to have the doctor assign me a new diet (which equated to a new Xeroxed copy of the old one). Or when grocery shopping, he still purchased only what he deemed "proper diet food." My mother, meanwhile, tried to threaten me by saying she wasn't going to buy me any new clothes and that when I grew out of my current size, I would be out of luck.

I knew I wasn't going to be walking around naked in two months. Their threats meant nothing to me. In fact, they taught me a wonderful lesson: Gaining weight makes the parents unhappy.

So screw you, Mom and Dad. I'm eating a box of Twinkies.

I was making daily trips to the grocery store just a couple of blocks from our house. I would come home with a full bag and immediately take it to my room. If Mom or Dad happened to be around, I would have to be careful to hide the food from them. This meant being stealth-like about the trash as well; I couldn't risk them discovering any empty junk food packaging. Luckily I was in charge of all the household chores.

High School Gregg's Typical Daily Binge

1 large pack of Nutter Butter Peanut Butter Sandwich Cookies

1 large pack of Chocolate Chip Cookies

6 cans of Snack Pack Chocolate Pudding

8 Hot Dogs (eaten raw or cooked)

8 slices of American Cheese

Ketchup, Mustard, Miracle Whip

1 gallon of Chocolate Ice Cream

6-pack of Coca-Cola

I was no longer stealing money to fund my habits. Instead, I was earning it by baby-sitting. I became quite good at it, and soon discovered that other families kept delicious foods in their houses all the time. I couldn't believe that families I baby-sat for put up with how much snacking I would do while watching their children.

I would wait for the kids to go to bed before I began my binge. By the time the parents came home, I'd be so stuffed that it was all I could do to not to buckle over in pain. And yet they had me back, time and time again.

Whenever I was too "hungry" to wait for the kids to go to bed, I would tell them we were going to play hide-and-seek. They would hide somewhere inside the apartment or house while I counted to 100 in the kitchen. While they scurried off, I'd begin stuffing myself with whatever food I could find. After a while, the kids would call out to me "Are you at 100 yet?"

"Not yet," I'd yell from the kitchen while chewing, as I continued to stuff my face.

There were families who, after a while, *did* stop calling for my baby-sitting services, as I was literally eating them out of house and home.

Soon I weighed over 275 pounds. My mom was miserable about my weight and embarrassed to be seen with me in public, which, lucky for her, was seldom.

I made my best attempts at preserving what little bit of self-esteem I had left. When getting dressed for school, I would ask Lori if I looked "FFAFK" (Foxy for a Fat Kid). I don't remember how that phrase came to be. I knew it was silly, especially given the old school use of "foxy," but my intent was earnest. I knew I was fat and that I couldn't wear the same kinds of clothes other kids did, but I still wanted to look my best.

"So, Lori, do I look *foxy for a fat kid?*"

"Yes," she'd always respond. Lori was one of my biggest fans.

Starting high school was scary. Ours was a big school with lots of students I didn't know. To make matters worse, I was a freshman, the lowest of the low within the armed forces high school system.

In one of my first classes, the teacher had us sit in a circle and share our future career goals with each other. Everyone took turns explaining how they wanted to be a doctor, architect, businessman— you name it.

When it was my turn, I leaned forward and proudly told the class I wanted to be a movie star—not an actor or someone working in show business, but a *movie star*.

The kids erupted into laughter and one remarked, "Forget star…he'll be a *planet.*" I had a difficult time remaining in that circle of students for twenty more minutes. The worst part was that the teacher didn't jump to my defense. But in hindsight, it probably wouldn't have helped.

I was forced to face facts. I was fat and unpopular.

LIGHTS, CAMERA, ATTRACTION

I knew I had to do something. I decided to parlay some of my baby-sitting riches into a home movie camera. I bought a cheap version, because I still wanted to have money left over to keep me in my grocery supplies.

What was I going to do with my new camera? Why, become the next Steven Spielberg, of course. I hatched a master plan. I was going to make a movie and cast the high school's most popular kids in all the roles. This would be my opportunity to click in. And guess what? It worked. It seems that if you cast a few star football players and their cheerleader girlfriends in your cinematic opus, you suddenly acquire a little respect. It didn't matter that these popular types weren't really my friends. The fact that I was getting face time with them meant something to my other classmates—especially to those who seemed repelled by me because of my excess weight.

My cinematic masterpieces were never truly recognized for their greatness. The subject matters? A twenty-minute feature documenting the lives of *Charlie's Angels* when they were still in high school, complete with their first crime to solve and a short movie about the exploits of Tabitha, the daughter from *Bewitched*, in high school. What can I say? I was a child obsessed with reruns.

I made several more movies over the next couple of years. Including a space adventure with the oh-so-original title of *The Third Encounter*, and a disco version of *The Wizard of Oz* titled *Discoz*. Since I lived in Germany, I had no idea that the similarly themed *The Wiz* already existed. I promise there's no need for a copyright infringement suit.

I cast my sister in several roles, as I always wanted her around me. We had lots of fun making movies. I would spend days editing them and then created musical soundtracks.

Neither my mom nor dad ever wanted to watch my celluloid creations. Whenever I announced that I wanted to be a filmmaker I would get in trouble. I guess they never saw me reaching such lofty goals and so didn't want to encourage them.

But it was thanks to the movie-making that I started developing some self-confidence—all despite my girth and shyness. My increasing popularity was further aided by my continued theater arts work. On stage I was boisterous, funny, and blessed with what I was told was an incredible tenor singing voice. Here was this huge kid with a "lovely" singing voice.

Opera, anyone?

Throughout high school, Lori never had a problem with her weight. But she did get the bad acne inherited from my father's gene pool. And while the wide-spanning ears I had as a toddler went "back" on their own, Lori's wide-spanning ears eventually had to be surgically pinned back.

About the same time that Lori got surgery to have her ears pinned back, my mom got her nose done for "medical reasons." She was continuing her morph into a hip, single chick who had all the guys crooning and swooning—or so she thought.

My mother could've given Cruella de Vil a lesson in depravity, but I had been brainwashed by her to see my dad as the reason we didn't have a normal childhood—I had been trained to see *him* as the enemy. I thought he was the reason for all the turmoil at home. Mom never hesitated to remind me that Dad was a drunk who was ruining his career and our family's reputation.

I didn't want to admit that my mom was getting quite a reputation of her own. Every now and then I would hear other kids in high school make comments; kids who had overheard their parents talking. Apparently my mother was the biggest flirt at the hospital. And her act was working with most men, especially the married ones.

Often she would stay away from home for days at a time, which was fine by Lori and me. Other times, she would call in the middle of the night to make an announcement.

I'd wake up and answer the phone, "Diana McBride's residence"— to find it was her calling from some bar, telling me she wanted me to sleep downstairs in the basement "maid's room." We were living in a third floor apartment and each apartment was assigned a small storage room in the basement that had previously been used for maids.

My protests were to no avail. Mom would scream at me to get down to the basement immediately because she was bringing someone home. She instructed me to bring my clothes and books for the next school day and that I should ring the doorbell in the morning, and pretend to be a neighbor's kid who was there to walk the dog.

What could I do? It was usually between 2:00 and 4:00 a.m., and I'd gather my clothes and head downstairs. Little did Mom know that I'd watch for her from the basement window. Sure enough, about twenty minutes later, she would walk by with some shadowy guy. It was generally a different man each time it happened.

The maid's room was a scary place to be. Since all of these small rooms were now used for storage, there was no one else residing on that level and it wasn't a secure area. I would hear lots of noises from the street. Or were they coming from the dimly lit hallway outside our maid's room door? I could never tell. And that unknown terrified me.

The very first time this scenario happened, I got so scared that I went back upstairs to our door to ring the doorbell. My mom answered the door, saw it was me and shut the door in my face. I just stood there, not knowing what to do.

Inside the apartment, I heard her and her man du jour talking. He asked who it was. I heard her tell him that it was "Just some neighbor kid I pay to walk the dog. He's here very early."

Yeah, it was very early—like 4:00 a.m. very early!

A moment later the door opened. My mom handed me the dog leash with Mac attached. I returned him after the walk in the same fashion.

Just some neighbor kid . . .

The next evening I was admonished for coming to the door at that hour. My mother told me never to let it happen again, and then went on to instruct me that when it was an appropriate time to walk the dog in the future, I should ring the doorbell from downstairs, outside the building, as if I really were a neighbor's kid and didn't have a key to the building.

"Okay," I told her. I didn't know what else to do.

There were times when she would have a steady man in her life and after a while I was allowed to sleep in the apartment. This situation wasn't much better.

Bernard, a young Frenchman, and my mom would disappear into her bedroom for wild bouts of noisy sex. One night I was awakened by loud, scary yelps. I got out of bed and pounded on my mom's bedroom door, convinced that Mac (who usually slept in my mom's room) was in the throes of a rabbit-chasing nightmare.

The yelps stopped. But it was then that I realized Mac was in the living room looking just as confused by the questionable sounds as I was. The errant sounds had been coming from my mother.

Yuck.

One more reason to detach sexually from society and myself. I later realized that my layers and layers of blubber were assisting me nicely with this particular objective.

CENTER STAGE

Lori and I had both become extremely active in community theater, and we were developing a following due to our singing voices. We appeared in several musicals and even received some glowing write-ups in local newspapers. Lori was being cast in lead or ingénue roles because of her "normal" size and beauty. And I was still relegated to the chorus or the occasional character role because of my size.

But even from the back of the chorus, I would sing loudly enough that people could hear me. It was immature of me, but at that time I just wanted to be heard, if not seen. I don't deny I'm a ham. That's a trait that always came naturally, despite my intense shyness and my conviction that *everyone* was judging me because of my size.

The best part of community theater was meeting and becoming friends with lots of different people. I always gravitated toward the adults in their twenties and thirties, as there were few teenagers in our productions.

One of my favorite friends was Vickie. She was a wild-eyed redhead who had all the guys crushing on her, even though she was happily married at the time. I baby-sat for her a lot and became good friends with her family.

On days that I would baby-sit for Vickie, I would go to her house early just to hang out or to have her cut my hair. She was a woman of many talents.

One day I sat in Vickie's kitchen as she cut my hair. We giggled and talked and giggled even more. I was relating stories of Massachusetts and Singapore. As I went further into the stories, I noticed that something was bothering Vickie. Her tone had changed and she suddenly seemed very concerned.

Soon she put down the scissors, sat in front of me and took my hand. "Gregg," she began, "it's okay. I know you're adopted. And I still love you anyway. You don't have to make up stories about your family and pretend anymore. We all know."

Adopted? I was anything but adopted.

I pleaded with Vickie to believe me, but my mom had once again done a terrific job of convincing everyone in our military community that I was adopted. The story went that she was too young to have had a high-school-aged son—she was lying about her age, too. I'm guessing at this point Lori was being claimed as my mom's actual child. But not me; I was still "adopted."

I was mortified after that. I didn't bring it up again. Everyone thought I was adopted. It was just a known "fact" within the community.

To this day, I don't think Vickie believed me when I told her I wasn't adopted.

The funny thing is, whenever anyone publicly attacked my mother because she was sleeping around with almost everyone in the community, I would jump to her defense. She had trained me all too well. It was my father I was supposed to hate. Not her.

Dad wasn't doing anything to help my skewed perspective. He was a drunk. Something people enjoyed gossiping about because of his high-ranking officer status; however, by then he was continually being passed over for promotion.

My dad would come by on Saturdays to do the grocery shopping. The spankings had stopped, usually because Mom wasn't around to report how "naughty" I was the previous week. Dad was usually in and out of there like a bullet.

Meanwhile, sparks of love were flying at the community theater.

We were in rehearsal for a musical theater show, *Purlie*, and there was someone in the chorus who caught my eye. She was thin and beautiful. Because she was wearing a scarf wrapped around her hair, I initially assumed she was some random housewife, but it turned out she was my age and attending the same high school.

Her name was Amy. And she liked me too. I thought she resembled the young Phoebe Cates—the actress from *Gremlins* and *Fast Times at Ridgemont High*—and I liked the fact that someone so pretty was interested in me.

Despite having other crushes on several popular girls, I soon asked Amy to be my girlfriend. We were together for quite a while by high school standards—much to the chagrin of her parents.

Amy's parents saw me as double trouble. First, because of my fat "problem," they could not understand how their daughter could be attracted to someone so big. Second, because Amy's father was a doctor at the military hospital and was all too familiar with my mom's dicey reputation.

Amy's parents also thought I was adopted and Amy would struggle to defend me to her overprotective parents. They felt I was lying about not being adopted and that I had conned Amy into believing the same.

Amy loved me. And I loved her. But my detachment from any sexuality left Amy with much to be desired. I just couldn't get close in that way. Even kissing and making out was difficult for me. Whether to chalk it up to the sexual abuse in my early childhood, my mom's accounts of Dad masturbating while looking at the Sears catalog, or my mom, herself, wailing like a banshee while having sex with her Frenchman, I was now officially afraid of any kind of intimacy.

I was too young to realize that this fear could have something to do with the layers of blubber I added to my body—almost a barrier of sorts that I worked to maintain through my constant eating.

Amy was patient, kind, and understanding. Even so, her affection was often put to the test. One night we went to the movies and I sat down next to her in my theater seat—only to have the seat instantly buckle and break from my excessive weight.

I was mortified. But true to form, I played it off as any class clown would. I looked to Amy and said loudly, "Amy, I can't believe you broke that seat."

I guess the tone of my voice was funny because people actually laughed *with* us. Amy wasn't angry at me for jokingly diverting the blame to her. But underneath my smile I was horrified. A horror I didn't share with Amy at the time. Even with her I needed to be the class clown. Being escorted to another pair of seats by the angry manager was not pleasant. But I kept a smile on my face the whole time and throughout the movie. Amy wasn't the wiser.

Amy remains fascinated by that incident to this day. And who can blame her? It's not every day you date someone with killer thighs . . .

Amy was also the one who tried to discuss my mom's reputation with me. She tried to help me admit out loud what I already knew deep down inside. I shared with Amy the stories about how my mom abused me, but I hated it when Amy would verbally attack her. I was embarrassed because I knew what a tramp Mom was, and her reputation around the hospital where Amy's father worked was sordid indeed.

One Christmas day, Amy joined my mother, my mother's boyfriend-of-the-moment, Ken, along with my sister and me for dinner. My mother had toiled all day on her festive dinner, a very rare occurrence, and the mood was jovial. True to form, Mom had prepped me and Lori with the day's lies—to be told for Ken's benefit.

Mom had prepared a magnificent turkey, but we were to lie and tell Ken it was goose because that was what she had promised to make for him. Before dinner, I had slipped to Amy that the main course was indeed turkey but that mum was the word.

Well, during dinner, Amy mentioned the "T" word and my mom choked on her saliva. Amy then talked about her and me being in high school together.

Oops. Too much information!

Within seconds, Amy and I were summoned to the kitchen and met with a menacing glare as Mom hissed through clenched teeth that we were not to verbally ruin her *special* dinner for Ken. Apparently Amy's "admission" that we were in high school played against whatever stories my mom had been telling Ken. And, believe it or not, I was mad at Amy and *not* my mother. In my fragile view of the world, Amy had ruined my closest shot at being like one of those pretend families on television, even if just for a moment.

I loved Amy but couldn't be there for her as a real boyfriend. It took everything in me to protect my self-esteem, which sometimes made me come off as a stuck-up person. Amy might argue that it wasn't just "sometimes."

Well, heck—wasn't I "foxy for a fat kid?"

After a while, my romance with Amy fizzled. Mainly because the romance aspect of our relationship had never really taken off. But we remained just as close, sharing the evil tales of both our wicked mothers. We nicknamed mine "Diana Doll" (the Barbie-like doll that comes complete with bleached hair, blue eye shadow, and spring-form legs).

We did have our fights; especially whenever Amy attacked my mom or even Lori. In my mind I still envisioned my family as *The Brady Bunch*. I wanted so badly to live up to that happy TV-family standard. With only one military-run channel that showed American TV in Germany, we were often exposed to reruns as opposed to the current TV fare that was airing in the United States. But my family never could live up to the Brady's—or any TV family's—standards. Amy saw this and tried to enlighten me. She saw my potential for depth. But I wanted to remain in the dark, literally, and eat contraband junk food while there.

COMING IN FOR A LANDING

One day my dad came to Lori and me with "exciting news." He had met a flight attendant from Scotland and they were going to live together. We couldn't have cared less and couldn't, for the life of us, figure out why he was telling us this.

We both stared back at him with blank faces. "So?"

Soon, Bonnie and my father were living together. She had quit her job with the airline and left her family in Scotland to live with my dad. I didn't know it at the time, but she and I weren't that many years apart in age.

Bonnie was nice enough, but she had a problem with the fact that my dad already had a family—not that she would have to worry, since my dad never really acknowledged his said family in any way.

Since the legal driving age in Germany was seventeen, there were still times that Lori and I needed my father to drive us to certain places. One Sunday afternoon, Dad had promised to drive us to the movie theater. He came to pick us up with Bonnie in tow. We were on our way to our destination when Bonnie burst into tears. Apparently, they had been at an afternoon party and then had to leave early so Dad could drive us to the movies.

Bonnie was hysterical over this, pleading with my father and asking when she wouldn't have to put up with his "abusive behavior" anymore. Lori and I were watching this drama unfold from the backseat of the car.

My father leaned over and said to Bonnie in a reassuring voice, "Soon these kids will be out of our lives. I promise."

I don't think my father realized then or to this day what it was that he said in front of my sister and me. While Bonnie tried to calm her tears, Lori and I held our breath until we arrived at the movie theater. Dad had been late picking us up, so we rushed inside after buying our tickets. We had to assure dad that we'd take a bus home—not that either my sister or I knew how to take a local bus in Germany. But neither of us wanted to get back in that car again.

Once inside the movie theater, Lori and I looked at each other and laughed. As I reflect on that event today I realize that it might appear to be an odd reaction, but I guess it was the only response that allowed us to continue with our lives and not completely lose our minds.

Soon after that Dad and Bonnie got engaged. She went home to Scotland to officially apply for her visa to live permanently in Germany. While Bonnie spent her last bit of time in Scotland, my father moved from their apartment into our buiding's maid's room. He wanted to save up his money so he and Bonnie could afford a nicer apartment once she came back.

Meanwhile, my ever-expanding girth was close to 300 pounds, but it didn't seem to be hurting my growing popularity. I was excelling in school, and had been accepted to the private college of my choice. I received several drama and solo singing awards in all-Germany-High-School competitions and continued to appear in local community theater productions to standing ovations. People especially enjoyed it when Lori's and my voice were paired together, such as when we played Roger and Jan in the stage musical *Grease*.

Our parents never attended our shows—neither high school nor community theater—and never shared in or even acknowledged our successes. We didn't care. We had done what we could to inoculate ourselves from the apathy and cruelty of our parents. Instead, we embraced the acceptance and love from the community.

The local press's terrific reviews of *Grease* came pouring in. Neither of us were in the leading roles, but Lori and I had still become the standouts in the show. As a result, a reporter interviewed me for a story that appeared on the front page of the local paper.

One night my mom's boyfriend, Ken, was sitting at the dining room table when I walked in. I said, "Hi," quickly trying to rush my bag full of groceries past him.

Ken asked me, "So . . . how does it feel to be in high school again?"

"What?" I asked.

Ken referred to the newspaper article about me, which mentioned my high school activities, and said that my mom had told him I was upset about the article since I was an adult going to college.

Ever the chameleon and quick on my feet, I covered my mother's lies adeptly by telling Ken that the reporter who interviewed me was German and may not have understood my answers since English was his second language. I then disappeared into my bedroom, unable to wait to attack the food in my grocery bag of comfort.

Later I found out that my coverage of Mom's lies wasn't as adept as I had thought. She was furious with me because Ken had become suspicious. She screamed at me at the top of her lungs, and ordered me to call Ken and tell him that I had purposely lied to the reporter.

I refused to do it.

Mom stuck her wicked-witch-of-a-finger in my face, waving it around while reminding me that she was "the boss" and if I didn't do what she said, then she would never let me be involved in any other community theater productions. I could hear Lori crying in her room as my mom and I fought. Mom went on to threaten my college and every other dream I held dear.

Enough was enough. I snapped. I shoved her pointing finger out of the way and rushed to the phone. I didn't know who to call. I was in a foreign country. So I called the military police.

A man answered the phone and I told him I was reporting an emergency. He asked what the nature of the emergency was.

Trying not to cry I said, "My sister and I are victims of child abuse."

"What kind?" he asked.

I was stumped. It had been a while since my last belt beating. How could I describe this current abuse? A long pause and then finally I replied, "Mental."

Another long pause, this time from the other end of the phone. No response, just dead air.

Then, clearing my throat, I gave him my name and address, but I could tell the call and the information exchange had been useless. Looking back I realize that it was a different era, and the military police operator didn't know how to process what I had described.

After I hung up the phone, I turned around to find my mother standing behind me, breathing fire. She told me to go down to the maid's room and "Get your father."

I headed down to the maid's room to find my dad out cold. It took me forever to wake him up. The stench of alcohol seeped through his pores as he tried several times to pull himself upright. His legs wobbled when he stood up, and then he stumbled as he made his way upstairs to our third-floor apartment. I cried and pleaded with him to take my side. He was disoriented and nothing I said seemed to be reaching him.

Once I finally got him into the apartment, Mom proceeded to tell him what I had done. "He gave them our address," she said in a panicked tone. My dad just stood there, bleary-eyed and dumbfounded.

After a moment I was ordered to go to my room and never to repeat that behavior.

As soon as I got to my room I searched for food. It was all gone. There was nothing there. Nothing to eat. Nothing to comfort me. Nothing to help me smash down my pain. Nothing for me to force-feed my sadness and hopelessness. My stomach felt like it was eating itself. I tried to cry some more—subconsciously I knew I needed to vent my fear and frustration. But, by then, my tears had dried up.

I've had a difficult time crying ever since.

The police never responded that evening. Or ever.

None of us spoke about that night again. But for the first time I began to realize what a true and utter *monster* my mother was. And that my father was a monster as well—for letting my mom get away with her abuse.

It's amazing that Lori and I excelled as much as we did in high school. We never had any encouragement from our parents. They weren't even around to make sure we *went* to school.

I never got involved with alcohol or other drugs while attending high school. There were many opportunities since the drinking age in Germany was much lower than in the United States, not to mention that no German bartender would bother to check IDs as long as you had the money to pay for whatever drink you were ordering. But my drug—or *libation*—of choice continued to be Twinkies and other delectable goodies instead.

Upon my high school graduation, I learned that my parents' four-year-long divorce proceedings were final. Along with this came another revelation. Over the years Lori and I and our parents had contributed to two different savings accounts—one for Lori's college education and one for my own. As far as my sister and I knew, these funds were available and earning interest to fund our higher education. Now it turned out my dad had spent most of the money on his drunken binges and attorneys fees to defend himself against the various DUI charges he'd faced.

This was my mom's explanation as to why both savings accounts were now defunct. My dad claimed it was used to pay for travel expenses. No matter the real reason, fact was the money was gone and Lori and I would now have to seek financial aid and student loans if we wanted to attend college.

It was the summer before college, and I was still determined to attend. I was equally determined to take off the weight and be thin, gorgeous, and loved (in that order) before I embarked on my journey of higher education.

Consequently, this became the summer when my sister and I discovered the marvel of diet drinks called Sego that were sold in the local military-operated grocery stores. With this over-the-counter liquid diet plan, you were to drink four twelve-ounce cans of "great-tasting" fluid a day (so great "you'll forget you're dieting!"). That was it. You were to consume nothing else.

The fact that my parents would let an eighteen-year-old boy and a fourteen-year-old girl go on such a harsh dieting regime boggles my mind today, but of course, neither of them was really around to put a stop to it. So long as it wasn't deemed "junk food," Dad would buy anything that was put on the weekly grocery list.

The Sego drinks turned out to be one of the first diets I was able to stick with. It was simple. There was no thought required and little temptation during meal preparation, which consisted of popping off an aluminum lid. For two whole months, Lori and I downed those chalky-tasting beverages in place of balanced meals. No chewing. Just drinking. I'm not sure why Lori even enlisted in such a program. She was hardly overweight. Perhaps it was moral support.

Despite an intake of less than 900 calories per day, I hardly lost any weight. My metabolism seemed to slow down to a virtual halt, all the while I was growing taller, inches-wise. But the inches around my belly remained.

Still, I stuck with the program.

The summer was uneventful by our family's standards. My mom traveled a lot with her boyfriend of the minute. It was at the Sego two-month mark that she and her current boy-toy showed up at our apartment, eating lunch.

That night, while I was throwing away my last can of Sego diet drink of the day, I found a half-eaten, crumpled up bag of Cool Ranch Doritos in the trash can. They were past their "enjoy by" date. My mother had thoughtlessly left the bag there, knowing Lori and I were on liquid diets and were trying to keep the apartment free of temptations. I stared into the trash can for about an hour.

And then . . . I reached into the trash, got my hands wet with various forms of garbage, grabbed the bag of Doritos, and ate the chips with abandon. They were stale and tasted like cardboard. Still, I devoured the whole remainder of the bag, sitting on the kitchen floor, feeling like Quasimodo who had snuck down from the bell tower.

I was never able to return to the confines of the liquid diet after that incident. My food intake went right back to cheese, cookies, and other high-fat foods. The little weight I had lost came back. Soon I shot up past 325 pounds.

At the end of the summer I was preparing to leave for college, and my mom and sister moved into a rented condominium situated closer to downtown Wiesbaden, outside of the military housing area. Neither parent was willing to travel to Florida with me to help me settle into college life—something they had promised to do, since I was nervous about living in the States again after being away for so long.

But I was on my own. Business as usual.

I weighed 335 pounds and I was nervous about traveling so far by myself. But as I boarded my flight for Florida everything besides those minor issues seemed right with the world.

Momentarily, that is.

ANOTHER PERSPECTIVE
ON GREGG AT THIS TIME

By Amy Wright-Israel, Gregg's High School Girlfriend

I'm not sure when exactly it hit me: I was dating the high school "fat kid." I don't deny that it was a little disconcerting to have classmates walk by and holler, "Skinny and Fatty!" when Gregg and I were walking together. But I wasn't after the popular vote, so I wasn't too fazed. Gregg had charisma. He made me laugh. He was indeed, as he liked to say, "Foxy for a fat kid." While I was shyer than shy he just seemed to have no fear. He would talk to anybody. Do anything. Even outrageous stuff. That got my attention.

My parents made the mistake of saying, "Well, somebody needs to love him. Look at him. Obviously he's miserable." I think I took that as a challenge.

Gregg? Miserable? If he was, he hid it well. He somehow managed to be popular and fun. I was actually jealous of him. He was also incredibly talented so we were in community theater, in honors chorus, and on the yearbook staff together. I think his sister hated me. His mother was straight up weird—pretending he was adopted and forcing me to uphold that lie if I ever spoke to her boyfriend. It was ridiculous, because they all seemed to look alike to me. Who was she kidding?

My dad worked at the same hospital where Gregg's mother worked and he would share rumors about her being the office "tramp." Her nickname around the hospital was "Passionata Von Climaxx." I was rather horrified.

"Dee-ahhhna"—as she insisted on being called at the hospital—pressured Gregg to lie about his age and say he was in his twenties. I sucked at lying. I screwed up at a dinner with her and her boyfriend and accidentally told the truth about us being in high school. That resulted in a trip to the kitchen for a stern lecture.

Gregg's mom had him terrified and forever jumping through hoops for her. There was nothing he wouldn't do. He would get on me for not playing along. I don't think I realized how evil she was really being to him. My own mom was very strict, and Gregg and I would commiserate and fantasize about sending our moms to the "island of bitches" so we could live a life free from both of them. We were teenagers.

Despite her strictness, my mom was normal compared to "Dee-ahhhna" and her bizarre fantasy world. I think her delusional lying warped Gregg's view of himself. Everything was about portraying an image. And it was all about lying, despite the elephant in the room: The elephant in the room often being Gregg.

Yes, Gregg really did break that damned movie theater seat and hollered out: "Amy, my God . . . I just can't take you anywhere!" It was funny and it was sad at the same time.

I remember how disturbing it was when I found Gregg devouring a gallon of ice cream that he'd taken from my parent's fridge. Back then I had no clue he treated food like a drug, and that he tried to numb himself by wrapping a wall of fat around his pain.

I had my own pain I was dealing with. My relationship with Gregg had always been a doomed love affair; for one, I wouldn't play snob and pretend to be something I wasn't. Gregg found the popular kids in high school for that. I couldn't understand why he needed their approval and would feel used and unloved as a result.

I also didn't understand his loyalty to his psychotic mother and to his sister. Fortunately, or unfortunately, Gregg had a confused perspective on what was going on around him. No matter how hard he tried, there was no denying the hell that was his world.

As our relationship developed, I became increasingly frustrated because I loved him. Every single pound of him. And I wanted him to love me. To really love me. I wanted him to notice me. But I was a pawn in his play for attention. I just refused to follow orders and didn't behave the way he hoped I would. For most of our time together, Gregg seemed most interested in being "popular."

After graduating high school, Gregg and I were in and out of touch over the years. We always find each other again as friends because of his damned sharp perspective and his blazing wit that can make me, literally, pee my pants.

I never would have thought that Gregg would fight his protective weight and take it all off and allow himself to be naked to this harsh world. Though I do remember when he once confessed how taken aback he was by something my father, a doctor, had said, "Fat people almost always die fat."

CHAPTER THREE

up, up, and a-weigh

Life as a young adult is trying for anyone. But imagine weighing over 300 pounds at eighteen years of age.

I was terrified of college. This represented more than just leaving home. It was also my first time back in the United States after living overseas for six-plus years. And again, neither of my parents accompanied me on my trip to begin my collegiate years.

The flight itself was harrowing, not because of any turbulence or other force of nature, that is unless you counted my massive belly as one.

Upon seating myself on the plane, I realized that the seat belt did not reach around my body because of my enormous stomach. I wasn't sure what to do. Should I tell a flight attendant? Should I get off the plane? I decided to strategically place a jacket over my lap to make it appear as though the seat belt was indeed fastened underneath. It was one of many little secrets I used to fool the world into thinking I was a normal size.

Or so I thought.

In South Florida I took an airport shuttle to Lynn University, a ritzy little private school in Boca Raton. The campus was immaculate, as were the bevy of model-like students. I scanned the crowd for anyone who might be bigger than I was. *Nada*. I was king of the fat kids. In fact, I was the *only* fat kid.

Florida's hot sun made matters worse. There's nothing more devastating than having to make your first attempt at looking cool in front of new people wearing Sears shorts and T-shirts for the "big and tall"—all while sweating profusely.

Let me tell you something. No one knows how to make clothes for the obese male. The crotches hang down at the knees and the polyester shirts hug every inch of a fleshy belly. The *Fashion Police* would have hauled me off had they been around at the time.

It was okay, though. I knew the tactic many overweight people adopt—become the class clown. I was given this opportunity in the school's theater program, which I was majoring in, and quickly got accepted in via my role as "the funny fat kid."

It was in Boca Raton that I implemented a brilliant plan: If you don't look like a model, hang around kids who *do*. I subconsciously sought out and befriended every "beautiful" person on campus. Little did I realize I was shunning the other "real-life" kids—in other words, I was doing to them exactly what I felt like everyone had always done to me.

I became friends with Kathi-Jo DeMilia and Doreen DeNigris— two of the most sought after beauties at school. This made me "cool" in everyone's eyes—especially my own. No one thought I could actually be dating either of those gorgeous ladies, but still, people wondered, "Why are those hot girls hanging out with *him?*"

I now had friends and earned accolades by standing out—in terms of talent and literally—in Lynn's theater program, but I still resorted to my secret food addiction when no one was looking. I maintained the same pattern I'd started with my parents, even though they were thousands of miles away. I *never* let anyone see me eat. Not breakfast. Not lunch. Not dinner. Not in-between meal snacks. Even though my meals were paid for as part of my tuition, and despite the fact that our campus was isolated and I didn't have a car, I never once ate at the college cafeteria.

Instead, I ordered food from the school's snack bar and took it back to my room and gorged myself, or I ordered from the local pizza delivery and did the same.

College Gregg's Typical Binge

1 large Italian Submarine Sandwich with Everything

1 large Philly-Style Cheese-Steak Sandwich

4 bags of Barbecue Potato Chips

3 large Lemonades

4 large Chocolate Chip Cookies

6 packs of Bubble Yum Watermelon Flavored Gum

My roommate, George, who was there on a student visa from Singapore, worked quite a bit and usually wasn't around. Whenever he was, I would take my food to a stall in the dormitory's giant communal bathroom. I wonder to this day if people using the bathroom realized where the smell of food was coming from. There I would sit—yes, on the toilet—stuffing food down my throat and using toilet paper for napkins. It was quite glamorous.

I was sure that no one knew I ate. I was convinced I was fooling everyone.

The ultimate milestone in making everyone realize I was "foxy for a fat kid" was when I became roommates with the best looking guy on campus, a model from Kentucky named Tom. At last, I thought, I was one of the beautiful people. And despite my delusional thinking, a strange thing occurred: With those new friends, I became surprisingly more active and even—*dare I say*—happy.

Then something even more surprising, something quite wonderful, happened. Without dieting, without monitoring my weight, without even consciously exercising, I began to shed weight.

I went from a 3XXX ("tent size" to the uninitiated) to a regular XL. For the first time in my life I was able to wear a Ralph Lauren polo shirt, the unofficial school uniform for any guy who deemed himself worthy at Lynn University.

Of course, Ralph Lauren polo shirts required major bucks, something I had little of. My mother rarely sent me money. I couldn't even afford shampoo most of the time. That's when I started shoplifting—from one manifestation of addiction to the next.

Committed to "fitting in" no matter what, I was determined to "own" some Ralph Lauren polo shirts of my own, and I did it the only way I knew how, via the "five finger discount." I'm not sure if that temporary bout of shoplifting was just immature kid stuff or another way of crying out for help.

Either way, help never came.

I thought I was happy. And in a way I was. Except for the times when I'd visit either of my parents. That was something I *had* to do because Lynn University, being a private college, would shut down for school breaks. No students were allowed to be on campus during those breaks, much less reside in the dorms.

My dad was now working as a civilian and living in Boston, married to Bonnie the flight attendant, who was pregnant with my half-sister, Nicole. Once Nicole was born, anytime during my visits when the four of us were out in public, people would assume that Bonnie and I were the couple and that Dad was the grandfather to my baby sister.

Dad was never thrilled with my visits, and Bonnie was even less excited. I was desperate to become a "member" of their family, but they wanted little to do with me.

One Thanksgiving break, Dad didn't want to pay for my transportation to Boston from Florida. He suggested that I hitchhike.

At first I thought Dad was joking around. When it became evident that he wasn't, I was horrified, given that hitchhiking 1,500 miles from South Florida to Boston would be pretty risky for all sorts of reasons. I wondered if my dad had even considered the danger involved. Whether he had or hadn't, his suggestion remained very unsettling.

Visiting my mom was even weirder. Lori had been suffering from Mom's direct abuse since I wasn't around to shield her anymore, and she had run away from home. I learned that Lori was eventually placed with a foster family in the greater Wiesbaden area in Germany.

The story my mother told was that Lori had turned to drugs and had become a terror to live with. Lori's version was more chilling; tales of my mother flying into uncontrollable rages and hunting Lori down when she would try to escape, at one point even attempting to run her down with a car.

Since I was staying with Mom while visiting, Lori chose not to see me, which I understood. But that meant it was just me, alone with my mom, which presented numerous challenges. The main one was that my mom continued to be embarrassed by my size. I had plateaued at XL and was now starting to gain weight again. Even if we were just running to the grocery store, she would suggest I not go, or if I did, she would want me to dress as nicely as possible, so as to look more "presentable."

Whenever we ran into someone she knew, she wouldn't introduce me.

I didn't care. For the most part we were getting along. I didn't mind corroborating her lies, like her continued lowering of her age over the summer, as long as she showed me a bit of affection from time to time.

And most of that affection came in the form of edible goods. She kept a full pantry of food for me whenever I was "home" in Germany during school breaks. It was as if she was willing to play along with my sickness as long as I was willing to play along with hers. I ate like a king. Actually, like a big fat king and his entire court. Forget ballooning back into a size 2XX. I was now bordering on 3XXX territory again. Don't let the "triple X" fool you. Nothing about my girth was sexy.

In the spring of my sophomore year at Lynn University my mother stopped writing, stopped calling, and stopped sending money. I was broke and started bouncing checks in order to get by. Finally, I called my dad to ask for help. I learned that he was sending my mom almost $300 per month for my individual, court-ordered child support. Only she wasn't sending me a cent of it. Thankfully, after checking with his divorce attorney, my father started funneling the settlement earmarked for my well-being directly to me.

My mother was furious and begged Dad to change his mind, telling him I would waste the money on drugs; apparently at that point both my sister and I were both drug addicts.

I will admit to being addicted, just not to drugs. Sure, I smoked a joint in college every now and then. I got my "first high" in the middle of a stage production—not a good thing, albeit a funny one. I got the giggles so bad I soon had everyone on stage laughing hysterically, all while in the middle of a "serious" play written by Mr. King, the head of the drama department, who wasn't the slightest bit amused by my villainous character coming down with a case of the giggles in the middle of Act I.

But even so, my addiction wasn't to drugs. It was to cheese, to pizza, to burgers, all eaten quietly while no one was looking. I would wait for my roommate to fall asleep in our tiny dorm room before partaking of snacks of any sorts. I would then take out the wrappers from the trash before dawn to hide all proof of my binge.

I put on even more weight. Was it being added to keep my parents away? If so, it worked. I was no longer invited "home" to Germany by my mom, and Bonnie wanted nothing to do with me, either. This meant my father also stopped inviting me to his place in Boston for school breaks.

There was just one problem: the campus would still close down, as did the dorms. So I began spending holidays and school breaks sleeping in public places like airports or bus terminals, or with the occasional kind soul who would let me sleep on the floor in their home. One such person was the head of the drama department, Mr. King.

I know this sounds so melodramatic, but I'm truly surprised I did not end up in more serious trouble with as many nights as I spent sleeping—or trying to sleep—in public places.

However, if the opportunity arose, I'd avoid sleeping in public places by becoming an intrusive guest to any Good Samaritan who had room on his or her living room floor for me to crash. This mostly equated to kindhearted teachers or college administrators (people I barely knew) since none of my friends at school lived locally and would return to their homes in other states whenever the campus was shut down.

STUDENT BODIES

When it was time to transfer up to Florida State University and I needed a rental car to transport my belongings, I had to ask the head of the athletic department to let me use her credit card in order to rent the car. I had no idea that you couldn't rent a car with just cash. I was stuck at the rental car lot without any other options.

Florida State University was an environment like no other. And Tallahassee was nothing like Boca Raton. Compared to Lynn University's easily accessible student population of 500, FSU touted over 22,000 students.

Finding the attractive people to befriend in order to fool the world, in my mind, into accepting me as a "normal person" was going to be difficult.

Initially, I thought I had lucked out when Tom (my great-looking roomie) and Kathi-Jo (one of the sought-after beauties) had transferred to FSU, as well. But both were quickly scooped up by fraternities and sororities, neither of which wanted anyone fat as a member.

It's humiliating to hear people mock your weight, sometimes when standing right next to you. Didn't they know that a human being lived beneath those layers of fat? Weren't they aware that a heart beat under the blubber? What that cruel Greek population at FSU couldn't see was how terribly small I felt despite my size. My armor of humor crumbled here as I tried to find my place in strange and unfriendly surroundings.

I was majoring in Communications with a minor in Theater, and so I thought I could make a decent impression with my old tricks of being the class clown with a decent singing voice. However, there were over 3,000 of us trying to get noticed within the FSU School of Theatre. The vehicle I was sure would allow me to get noticed in a good way was the school's Mainstage production of *The Boy Friend*. For the first time, I found the auditioning process daunting.

I needed a standout role in order to "win over" the audience as well as my new classmates, but most of the roles in that musical were for fit young men. Those weighing in at just under 400 pounds need not apply. I was fortunate to get cast in the small role of the Garçon (the waiter), an honor given the amount of people who were auditioning and my being new in the program, I was told.

How was I going to make an impression with only five minutes of stage time?

None of the cool kids in the theater department wanted anything to do with me. There were other class clowns already taking center stage—thin and attractive class clowns.

Being depressed about my weight, I did the only thing I knew how to do . . . *eat*.

I sat in my room and counted the minutes until 4:00 p.m. every day, when the local pizza and sandwich delivery places started delivering to the campus (heaven forbid I walk to any of those places). Every day at 4:01 p.m., I would order a truckload of food.

I'd make sure to order enough food for four, and also enough drinks for four—thinking the delivery driver would then assume it wasn't all for me—as if the delivery drivers cared. I put on more weight very quickly.

How quickly? I soon weighed over 400 pounds. The only clothes that fit were two pairs of sweat pants and a couple of oversized shirts. The sweat pants were awful, but nobody made jeans in my size.

Dormitory Gregg's Typical Binge

1 large Pizza with Everything

1 large Italian Hoagie with Everything

1 large bag of Barbecue Potato Chips

A variety of Candy Bars from the vending machines

1 large carton of Chocolate Milk

6-pack of Pepsi

I was now so fat my penis was literally retracted into my pelvis (due to my enormous stomach that engulfed my groin). I resorted to stuffing a sock or two into my crotch so the world would know I was male. I also maintained the beard I had grown during my last year at Lynn University.

I tried desperately to be "foxy for a fat kid," but it wasn't working anymore. I was huge. I was sweaty. I felt ugly. Therefore I *was* ugly. At least in my mind.

After six months I managed to land a "beautiful-person" friend in Tallahassee. She was a short, voluptuous bombshell named

Elizabeth, with big brown hair, big blue eyes, and big, curvy breasts. Bigger than my big "man" breasts, in fact. Men would walk into walls staring at her chest.

Elizabeth had the personality of a saint and a maniac rolled into one. She was never embarrassed to be seen with me; I knew people were impressed when they saw me with her. Despite my initial selfish reason for befriending her, a genuine friendship blossomed between us.

But I continued to eat. Oh sure, I *tried* to diet. For about eight hours every Monday. And sometimes on Tuesday. Often on Wednesday. Never on Thursday, Friday, Saturday, or Sunday, though. That was too close to the following Monday, any dieter's favorite day to "start." I tried every diet known at the time—multiple times.

College-Aged Gregg's Attempted Diet Plans

The Atkins Diet

Ayds Reducing Plan Vitamin and Mineral Candy

The Cabbage Soup Diet

Dexatrim

Diet Pills (both prescribed and over-the-counter)

The Grapefruit Diet

Optifast

The Rice Diet

The Scarsdale Diet

Slim-Fast

I even went to Overeaters Anonymous a few times, but found the small group of people were too familiar with each other and that I, as an outsider, wasn't really welcome. Today I know that was my reflection on one particular group and that I could have tried another group at another meeting time or day. But I didn't.

No matter what diet I began, regardless of the day I began it, after about eight hours I'd drive up to a drive-through window in my used Chevy Chevette and order enough food for a medium-sized family.

Then I'd return to my private living space where I would force the food down until it hurt. If there was anything left over, I would throw it away, convinced I would successfully begin my diet the following day.

Gregg's Typical Drive-Through Binge

MENU I

2 Quarter Pounders

1 Big Mac with extra Sauce

1 Filet-O-Fish Sandwich (to eat in the car on the way home)

2 large French Fries

1 box Mini Chocolate Chip Cookies

2 large Chocolate Shakes

4 Diet Cokes

MENU II

2 Double-Patty Whoppers with Extra Mayonnaise

2 large orders of Onion Rings

1 large order of French Fries

1 Chicken Sandwich

1 regular Cheeseburger (to eat in the car on the way home)

2 Chocolate Shakes

4 Diet Cokes

MENU III

1 whole Barbecued Chicken

1 large order Barbecued Spare Ribs

1 large order of Mashed Potatoes

1 large order of Biscuits

1 large order of Coleslaw

3 pieces of Mud Pie

4 Diet Cokes

I found that Elizabeth had an addiction, too, just not to food, though we joked that our version of sex was sharing the chocolate fudge cake at Jerry's Diner.

Elizabeth's addiction was to committed men. Whether it was the married, engaged, or simply having a steady girlfriend, these committed men would constantly turn their attention to her; and Elizabeth found this attention difficult to resist. Between my obesity and her dalliances we often found ourselves very alone. Luckily we got to spend that "alone time" together.

Elizabeth was a truly kindhearted soul. And she had a roommate, Gwen, who was very obese. Like me, Gwen was constantly dieting and bingeing and she was also the "funny girl." Once she tried to join the Navy because she liked their uniforms. I guess she didn't realize white garments weren't the best fashion choice for the normal-size-challenged.

The Navy wouldn't let Gwen join because of her weight.

Elizabeth, Gwen, and I became quite the threesome. As a member of this jolly trio I was looking forward to the time my mom's boyfriend-of-the-minute, John, was coming to town to visit me for a few days. I decided the four of us would go out for dinner.

Little did I know that all through dinner, John was coming onto Elizabeth by playing "footsie" under the table and that he even propositioned her later that night over the phone. Elizabeth hadn't wanted to tell me—but she finally did.

I was disgusted with John. But it got worse.

The next day, John and I were at brunch by ourselves. I was not bringing up the fact that I knew he was making passes at Elizabeth, but in an attempt to make him uncomfortable, I kept the topic of conversation on my mom.

Only my strategy backfired when the discomfort turned out to be my own thanks to John talking about how my mom loved me just like I was her own child—as if I weren't adopted.

I couldn't believe it. My mom was *still* telling people I wasn't her real son. I pretended that I suddenly felt ill and told John that I had to leave the restaurant. As soon as I was alone, I called Elizabeth. She consoled me as best she could.

Later that night Elizabeth and I got together, *over dinner*, to discuss the problems with my mother, my belly, and Elizabeth's love life.

Meanwhile, Gwen, who was nowhere near as large as I was, still struggled with her weight, and finally announced that she was going to take drastic measures and have her stomach stapled.

Everyone in Gwen's life, including Elizabeth, thought it was a wonderful idea. I was the only one who didn't. I felt like it was unnatural to have a metal puncture put into your stomach in order to stop eating so much.

Gwen *did* lose weight after having her stomach stapled, but it was through a violently gross process. In spite of the staple, she tried to eat as much as she always had, and ended up throwing up night after night. Every time I talked to Elizabeth, Gwen would either be on her way to, or just finishing, throwing up.

In my opinion the staple was no cure; it was a hindrance. Gwen wasn't really losing the weight; she was getting rid of it temporarily through artificial means. Sadly, she eventually gained the weight back. Despite my obesity, I knew that wasn't how I wanted to get rid of my weight.

I kept trying all the fad diets. You name it, I tried it. I'd wake up with the best of intentions, but always falter at some point during the day, sometimes as late as 11:00 p.m. I could never complete a full day of dieting, no matter how hard I tried.

And my weight was increasing rapidly. So much so that even my car, a trusty used Chevy Chevette, was showing wear and tear from my girth. The driver's side arm rest slanted upward after months of my left thigh pressing up against it while I drove. Even crazier, the floorboard of my car had worn through—think Fred Flintstone. When driving, you could see the street underneath the gas and brake pedals. I'm not sure if it really was the tremendous weight I would put onto the floorboard when getting in and out of the car. A friend suggested it might be salt from Florida's ocean air that was wearing it out. Only Tallahassee is about three hours from both Florida's east and west coasts.

My sweatpants were tighter around my waist, thighs, and calves than ever before. I had to replace them often, as the thighs would rub out and get holes after just wearing them three to four times. Finding clothes was getting to be impossible.

Along with the never-ending search for clothes that fit, I was also continually on the hunt for another "pretty female friend who would fool the world into thinking I was normal" of the moment. Thankfully, these "beautiful people" often came with beautiful personalities. This was especially true of my friend Erika, who I'd met when I first transferred to FSU and then connected with again when we were both auditioning for a college news program. I would always try and keep up my ruse of being hilariously unaffected by my weight when around others. But sometimes my two worlds would collide. One such time was when Erika and I were in a campus bookstore. Hanging from the ceiling was a grossly oversized FSU tee. The sign near the oversized T-shirt mockingly promised:

IF YOU FIT INTO THIS, IT'S YOURS!

Guess what? I had the store manager pull the shirt down. Then I tried it on. It fit perfectly. And this shirt was huge. Erika was amazed that I had the courage to go through the "fitting" in front of flabbergasted shoppers and the baffled store manager. Personally, I knew I had no choice. I needed the shirt. I had gotten so large that I truly had hardly anything left to wear.

At that point I stopped weighing myself. I couldn't have done it even if I had wanted to. Despite investing in an expensive electronic scale, the scale did not go up past 400 pounds. It would read "ERR" (for "error") whenever I stood on it.

Error? Really? Apparently so.

Even though I was faced with being clothes-less and dealing with a scale that couldn't compute, I still tried to lose weight, sure that getting rid of my blubber was key to my life's dreams of being liked, falling in love, and living out my Hollywood fantasy of being an actor, writer, and director.

My father never wanted to see me, but he still sent me money and encouraged me to see a doctor and inquire about the Optifast weight reduction program. I went to the doctor and weighed in. I was stunned. 464 and "0.5" pounds. I was mortified at the sight of all those numbers. I couldn't face the doctor. He was young and in-shape, not at all like the "older doctors" I'd mostly encountered up to that point. I felt less-than-human to be *that* heavy.

I looked down at the floor as the echo of "464.5 pounds" reverberated in my head. Then I noticed the doctor wasn't saying anything. I looked up and saw he was crying. He clenched my chart in his hands. Finally, he shared how terrible it made him feel to see someone so young facing such morbidly dangerous health problems.

I found myself reaching out and patting the doctor on the shoulder to console him, promising him that I would lose weight, and that he didn't have to worry.

Of course, right after the appointment I headed to the nearest grocery store, where I purchased the ingredients for a binge-fest.

Gregg's Typical Tallahassee Grocery Store Binge

3 pounds of Raw Hamburger

1 package of Hamburger Buns

Miracle Whip, Mustard, Ketchup

Onions, Tomatoes, Lettuce

Ready-To-Bake French Fries

1 gallon of Vanilla Ice Cream

Whipped Cream

1 jar of Chocolate Fudge Sauce

2-liter bottle of Diet Coke

I got home and cooked up a feast.

While that doctor was a stranger, it freaked me out that he was worried about my weight to the point of tears. It scared the hell out of me that someone actually cared about my health. I wasn't used to that kind of concern—from *anyone* in my life.

I gorged myself with the food I'd prepared, stuffing down all the fears, all the emotions, all the desires that made me want to be thin. I knew what being fat was about. I knew what it was like to feel like my stomach would burst. At times I was surprised it didn't. I knew how to squash the pain with Oreos or feed the loneliness with chips and ice cream. If I could get others to laugh at me or the embarrassing missteps that being so fat caused me to take, then they wouldn't see the sadness that wrapped around me like a pair of pants that were way too tight.

APARTMENT COMPLEX

I was now living off campus, in my own small studio apartment. Just me and Shadow, my cat that I adopted via animal rescue after seeing her little squinty-eyed face. We took one look at each other and knew it was love. The unconditional love Shadow offered felt so good; however, it wasn't enough love to dissuade my eating habits. The binges continued.

My studio apartment had a window air conditioning unit, but most days the place was still like a furnace thanks to Tallahassee's oppressive heat. But that didn't matter to me. There I stood in front of my stove, wearing a bulky brown terry cloth robe, sweating profusely as I fried up burgers or whatever else I was preparing to gorge on.

After my binges I would lay on my bed, desperately wishing for the air conditioner to kick-in and cool off my blubber-covered body. It was a horrific sight—one even I couldn't look at in my own mirror. At least Shadow didn't have a problem with my appearance, though her love proved to be of little comfort.

And yet, between classes, between being lonely and the bingeing, I honestly still tried to diet.

Honestly—I did.

Anytime I saw a magazine article that offered new hope in the form of a new diet, I'd buy it and try it. But by 10:00 a.m., I was reaching for chocolate or heading to a vending machine between classes. I never would get just one candy bar, rather, it'd have to be two or three. And I'd eat them in some dirty bathroom stall, sure that the world had no idea I weighed 464.5 pounds.

Despite my weight, there were times when I became the object of attention from young women who would call to profess their love to me. True story.

That happened while I was working as an overnight DJ for the local Top-40 radio station in Tallahassee, Gulf 104 FM. I'd been lucky to meet some people at a party who worked at the station, and when they discovered my penchant for creating different voices (thanks to my training pretending to be the female maid for my mom), they invited me in to audition for a DJ position.

Under the on-air name of "Greg Adams," I spun the hits, made silly jokes, and even called into other DJs' shows during their shifts at the station to vocally play different characters. On weekend nights I had the airwaves to myself, which is when I would get calls from various female listeners who would ask me if I knew how "sexy" I sounded on the radio.

Admittedly, I wasn't too surprised by that. I knew to lean away from the microphone when I ran out of breath introducing a song, which I always did. And I knew how to put on a more seductive tone when introducing some of the slower jams. Still, getting those calls provided a temporary boost to my ego, until the respective ladies would ask to meet me in person.

Enter the glitch. I knew there was no way those callers expected "Greg Adams" to weigh over 450 pounds. So obviously I could never let them see the real me.

I relied on the lame excuse that we DJs weren't allowed to meet any of our listeners; it was against station policy. But every now and then I would notice people outside the DJ booth window, which was accessible from the radio station's parking lot, trying to catch a glimpse of me. Since the DJ booth was soundproof, I could never hear anyone's reaction. But one time a female fan called back in, saying, "You never told me you weighed, like, a thousand pounds."

Nice.

Since all listener calls were screened and recorded *before* they went on the air, that remark never went public. But it had already hit, and wounded, its intended target.

That's okay though. There was comfort and acceptance waiting in whatever meal I would partake in right after leaving the radio station—even at 6:00 a.m., when my overnight weekend shifts were finished and I would head to a twenty-four-hour grocery store.

WHAT'S IN STORE

While they generally offered me a haven of comfort, my single most horrific moment as a fat man happened to me at a grocery store. I was a senior in college at the time, and it was just a couple of months before graduation. I had to be well over 464.5 pounds.

As I pushed my cart through the clean, bright aisles I filled it up with ingredients that would have me in severe pain later that night. But, oh, those first forty-five minutes of eating were going to be worth it.

That particular evening, I found myself in one aisle that was very crowded. It was the cereal aisle and I was picking out one "healthy" and one "unhealthy" cereal. When turning my cart to leave the aisle, I saw a bunch of shoppers on one end of the aisle.

Abort mission!

I quickly turned my cart toward the opposite end of the aisle, mortified to see it was just as crowded.

Why must everyone like cereal as much as me? I wondered.

Then I swallowed hard and looked down since eye contact with any stranger seeing my girth was forbidden, and pushed my cart toward the end of the aisle. At one point I passed a mom and her daughter. The little girl, who must have been around six or seven years old, made eye contact with me. There she was—a sweet, innocent cereal lover. So I risked everything and smiled at her. She stared back blankly. I continued past her and her mom, but as I did, she screamed out, "Mommy! Mommy! Why does that man have boobs?"

Oh. My. God.

Everyone—and I mean *everyone*—in that crowded aisle turned to look at the man with boobs. I was still sporting facial hair at the time, so there was no denying I was male. I quickly made my way down the aisle, holding my breath while my hands gripped the cart, determined to slink away before every shopper saw my 44Bs. Or were they Double Ds?

After rounding the corner I abandoned the cart and left the market, getting into my Chevy Chevette and racing away like a vampire fearing dawn's first light. Once safe in my apartment, I wished I had said something mean to the little girl—something that would have kept her up at night or, at the very least, made her pee her pants in front of all the other shoppers. I never did see her or her mother again.

On the way home from the grocery store that night, I stopped by a drugstore and bought several packages of over-the-counter sleeping pills. I decided I would take the sleeping pills and end my life after the following night's binge. I couldn't stand living in my huge body—or living with man boobs—any longer.

The next night, after a more clandestine grocery gathering trip, I cooked and toiled over the stove. Then I ate and ate and ate. After dinner I washed the dishes and took out the trash. I was cleaning up for reasons other than the idea of starting a diet the next day. I was cleaning up to clean up. I didn't want whoever discovered my body to know I had binged.

After all evidence of my binge was erased, I reached for the sleeping pills and began to pull them from their individual foil compartments. I was really going to do it. Since I couldn't seem to stop myself from bingeing, I was ready to have the pills do what I couldn't do. I was going to take my own life.

Just as I filled a glass with Diet Coke to take the pills, my cat Shadow, jumped up onto the bed. Shadow. The cat that loved me no matter what. No matter my size. No matter if I weighed 464.5 pounds or 475.

I pondered how it would take days before anyone would realize I was missing, and then possibly weeks before anyone would have investigated my apartment. I knew Shadow wouldn't be able to survive. So yes, that cat literally saved my life. I shoved the pills aside and never took them. Instead, I hugged my purring cat.

Thank you, Shadow.

Graduation was fast approaching. I was at my largest size ever. Deep down I knew I must have weighed around 470 pounds, but I wasn't willing to admit it or get near a scale that would show it. I didn't even know if doctor's scales went that high.

Despite my girth, I had basically excelled in college. I wrote and directed two feature-length student films, both of which played at local movie theaters and on local television. So while I was usually hiding from the world, I decided that attending my college graduation was important to me.

My parents, on the other hand, couldn't have cared less. Neither was interested in seeing me accept my diploma. At the time Dad was even living in the state of Florida, having moved there after Bonnie, a burgeoning agoraphobic, had decided she hated Boston and they had to move.

While talking to him one Saturday, Dad told me he couldn't attend my graduation—on a Sunday, the next day—because Bonnie was sick. Later I found out they were car shopping on the day of my graduation. I guess car shopping was good for Bonnie's flu symptoms.

I was *huge* walking across that stage to get my diploma. The entire graduating class's list of names and majors could have been projected across my girth. My graduation gown could have clothed half of a Third World country.

I was so mortified. So ashamed. So embarrassed. So *fat*.

Add to that the fact that while walking across the stage I actually became winded.

Was this it? Was I so huge that I was about to suffer the ill-health problems that the doctor had been crying about?

I remember my graduation photograph. You can't tell where my body ends and where the stage and auditorium begin. I was like a small planet moving across the stage. Turns out that kid who had mocked my wanting to be a "movie star" in high school was right; I had become a planet instead of a movie star.

It took everything I had to fake my smile as I accepted my diploma. I was getting worse and worse at making public appearances, convinced that I was being judged for every excess pound, and let's not forget that ever looming and haunting half-pound.

Here I was at the dawn of my adult life, once again wishing I could really end it somehow. I just had to make sure Shadow would be okay first.

ANOTHER PERSPECTIVE ON GREGG AT THIS TIME

By Kathleen (Kathi-Jo) Demilia-Gaudin, Gregg's College Friend

When Gregg and I talk about the past and he mentions his weight and how difficult it was for him in college, I find myself scratching my head. I don't remember Gregg as being "fat." Was he big? Yes. I remember hugging him at one time and not being able to fit my arms around him. But still, my memories of Gregg are not of the "fat guy," but rather of my very funny, very talented friend.

Gregg and I met as freshmen at Lynn University in Boca Raton, Florida. We were in almost all of the same classes and saw one another daily, but only got to know each other well when, one day, our English professor asked us to stay after class to discuss the papers we had recently turned in. I recall looking at Gregg and whispering, "Why do you think he wants to talk to us?"

Frozen with fear, I was looking to this relative stranger for some sort of reassurance, but Gregg shrugged his shoulders and winced, as if to say, "I'm as freaked out as you are!"

Did we do something wrong? I wondered.

It turned out our fears were unfounded as the professor asked us to stay after class because he was so impressed with our writing that he wanted to single us out and let us know that he would be expecting great things from us as the semester continued. The walk back to our dorms Gregg and I shared after that meeting resulted in a bond that has stayed strong ever since.

As time went on, Gregg and I came to recognize each other as true friends and we began to spend much more time together. We spent many a night talking about our romantic interests at the time or simply rehashing the plots of our favorite television series.

Thinking back on that era, I realize now that much of our time was spent over food. Gregg's roommate, Tom, had a car—and cars were in short supply at school at the time. The opportunity to go off campus was a huge draw for us, especially to pick up food.

Gregg would tell Tom that he needed to borrow his car to take me to go get shampoo. Now I did have very, very long hair and might have used more shampoo than most, but the idea that I was in need of a new bottle every two days should have raised at least an eyebrow, even for a college-aged boy. But Tom never questioned our excursions, and so off we went for subs or pizza or burgers—and then we'd spend time in the parked car, eating and listening to the radio, all while plotting how we would finally win the hearts of our secret loves.

When we moved on to Florida State, food was still a big part of our lives. We would sit in my dorm room waiting until 4:00 p.m. so we could call a local pizza place to have pizza delivered. We were too lazy to walk a few hundred yards to get it ourselves. Of course, Gregg would eat much greater portions than me and consume a lot more Diet Coke, but I never really thought about it. To me, Gregg was Gregg.

While Gregg has often talked to me about how shy he was, I honestly never noticed that myself. I've always known Gregg to be the life of the party—the resident comedian in the crowd. In fact, there were people I knew who didn't like to be around Gregg because of all the attention he got wherever he went. I'm not sure Gregg realized this at the time.

Many of Gregg's jokes poked fun at himself and his weight, and he was always able to put people at ease. I realize now that it must have been difficult for a man topping the scale at 400 or more pounds to audition for a Mainstage production at a school such as Florida State. But Gregg not only auditioned for the show, he got a role.

As Gregg grew larger, he got more secretive about his eating. He told me when he ordered food he would pretend it was for a group of people instead of just for him. Expressing this shame to me was painful for him and I don't think I realized the extent of it until much later.

Gregg mentioned that he felt as though I was embarrassed to be seen with him because of his size, but I truly don't remember feeling that way. I never thought of Gregg as fat. He was my friend—my best friend—and he was always there for me. He was probably the only person in my life who truly knew me as I was and not just the way I wanted people to see me, and I was probably one of the few people who knew him for who he truly was as well.

ANOTHER PERSPECTIVE
ON GREGG AT THIS TIME

By Erika Hamburg-Brown, Gregg's College Buddy

I first saw Gregg backstage at an FSU School of Theatre Mainstage production of *The Boy Friend*. He had a small part, which was a real coup for those of us just beginning in the theater program, and I was working for my stagecraft class. Gregg was always surrounded by laughing theater types.

A year or so later, Gregg and I met while auditioning for on-camera reporter roles for the FSU School of Communications' weekly news program *1600 Seconds*. Gregg was auditioning to be the movie critic and I was auditioning for an anchor position. I was a nervous wreck and a jabbering mess. To ease my nerves, I turned to him and began blathering on about my anxiety and subsequent diarrhea. It was then and there that our friendship was born.

My first impressions of Gregg were that he was funny and easy to talk to. His knowledge of film history and film production was amazing. He was writing, directing, and producing his own student films and getting them shown at local theaters. He projected such capability and confidence that I was a little in awe of his talent. His self-deprecating sense of humor signaled that I could say anything, confide anything, or be anything and never feel judged. My secrets were safe with him.

We shared meals from time to time at the local all-you-can-eat buffet or greasy spoon, and when I tell you he never ate more than one average plateful, I'm not lying. I loved spending time with Gregg. There was no drama, no romantic entanglements, and no peer pressure. We were always just two friends making each other laugh. A typical outing with Gregg might include sharing a bagel and coffee at The Annex (a snack shop next to the campus bookstore), where we'd make up ridiculously funny lyrics to songs, commiserate about our lives, and routinely re-imagine our futures as characters from one of the more recent feature films.

On one such day we walked into Bill's, the campus bookstore, to pick up some school supplies and we both noticed this huge FSU T-shirt hanging from the ceiling. The sign said something like "If it fits you, it's yours." The shirt was beyond immense, hanging from the ceiling like a billboard sign. Gregg said he thought it would fit him. I told him it was way too big and started searching the T-shirt shelves for something I thought might be more his size, but he said his size wasn't there. I saw a 2XX and a 3XXX but he kept shaking his head "No." *What size was he,* I wondered?

I never asked Gregg about his weight or his eating habits or anything like that. We never talked about that kind of stuff.

Gregg said, "I wanna try it on—I could get a free shirt!" I was amazed at his courage; first, that he called over the manager to take the shirt down from the ceiling; second, that he tried it on in front of everyone; and third, that when it *did* fit, he didn't appear to be upset. I don't think the store manager thought he would ever have such a customer when he originally hung the shirt with that sign. He looked shocked and was at a loss for words. He said, "Well . . . um . . . I guess you can have it!" Gregg thanked him and, keeping the new T-shirt on and holding his old shirt over his arm, we walked out of the store laughing.

At the time I assumed Gregg was comfortable in his body and accepting of his size. Honestly, I found that trait extremely admirable. I remember feeling anxious during the T-shirt incident because I was afraid someone was going to say something cruel to him. I was afraid someone was going to make my dear friend feel badly. Little did I know this was exactly what had been happening to Gregg since he was a child. Gregg had shared only bits and pieces of his life story with me— his father's ineptitude at showing compassion and his mother's cruel and psychotic behavior. In spite of all of that, the last thing Gregg ever wanted to be seen as was a victim.

AGE	WEIGHT
18	325/335 lbs.
20	400 lbs.
22	464 lbs.
23	457.5 lbs.
27	450 lbs.
28	435 lbs.
29	185 lbs.
30	285 lbs.
30	185 lbs.

PART II

during

CHAPTER FOUR

never say die(t)

The real world. The real thing. The real me.

Strike that.

The last thing I wanted to get in touch with after graduating from college was the *real* me. I weighed well over 450 pounds and had exactly one pair of stretched-out sweat pants and two oversized T-shirts to wear and nothing else—with the exception of my big brown terry cloth robe that could double as a blanket for a California King-sized bed.

I was huge. Just answering the phone made me run out of breath. Crouching down to get into my car, the one with the hole in the floorboard, caused my heart to beat faster. Being seen in public was more than I could handle, mentally.

There were very few times I'd venture out for reasons other than work or food.

One rare exception I remember is of teaching water aerobics (yes, you read that correctly)—or should I say *my* version of water aerobics—to my friends Elizabeth and Donald. It was around midnight on a hot

Tallahassee summer night. I put on the boom box and "taught" class to my two friends who, for some reason, humored me. We laugh about that to this day.

There I was, weighing over 450 pounds, in the pool with my shirt off. The veil of darkness helped me feel more comfortable— plus Elizabeth and Donald were more than willing to gyrate to my watery moves while listening to the groovy beats of hit songs from the 1980s. Perhaps the fact that this took place after midnight and that no one else was around was the reason I was able to do it.

It's interesting that I felt comfortable enough to do something like that on one very random occasion, yet in day-to-day living I barely had the courage to look at myself in the mirror much less let the public catch a glimpse of me. Beyond that single water aerobics outing I do not recall getting out of the apartment for social reasons at all during that time.

Any overweight person knows that walking out in public with excess poundage can be a devastating experience requiring extreme courage. Whenever I walked down the street, I felt I became the butt of all jokes, the focus of all cut-downs, and the target of all laughter. Likely this wasn't always the case, but often it was. And as a result I was becoming a literal shut-in.

I convinced my dad I was applying to different graduate schools in order to further my education beyond my bachelor's degree. The truth was that I did fill out a few forms, but any calls I made were to local fast food places that delivered. I could exist in my apartment without ever having to venture into public.

Looking back now, I realize that becoming a social shut-in is the worst thing an overweight person can do. I was no longer surrounded by people I knew. In fact, I was no longer surrounded by people *at all*. The only "people" I was regularly coming into contact with were the images of trim, slim beautiful people who came to me via my television set. It was a most unrealistic view of the world, and one I compared myself to with great persecution.

Beyond not wanting to put myself "out there" for ridicule, another reason for becoming a shut-in was to make sure no one would ever see me eating. I still thought that if people didn't see the food entering my mouth, they wouldn't know I was a gluttonous pig.

My MO was almost always the same. I would order several pizzas, sandwiches, pasta dinners—you name it—and have them delivered whenever possible. Often I'd order from more than one restaurant on the same evening because I'd want a variety of foods to consume. My newly acquired post-college credit cards were footing the bill.

And boy, did I continue to think I had the food delivery drivers fooled. When the driver came to the door, I'd yell out "I'll get it, Kathi-Jo" to my cat, before answering the door. I figured that way the driver wouldn't assume I was going to eat the food all by myself. Great plan, huh? (*As if the driver even cared.*)

Gregg's Typical Delivery Binge

MENU I

4 pieces Fried Chicken

1 pound of Barbecued Ribs

1 large order of French Fries

1 large order of Onion Rings

1 large Grilled Chicken Sandwich

Extra Ketchup and Sauces

3 pieces of Apple Pie A-La-Mode

4 Diet Cokes

MENU II

1 large order of Sweet & Sour Chicken

1 large Pork Egg Roll

1 large order of Cashew Chicken

1 large order of Fried Rice with Pork

Extra Sauce

1 extra order of Fortune Cookies

6 Diet Cokes

MENU III

1 medium Pepperoni Pizza

1 medium Deep Dish Hamburger Pizza

1 large Italian Submarine Sandwich

2 bags of Potato Chips

4 slices of Raspberry Cheesecake

4 large Diet Cokes

Once I had the food I'd put on my brown terry cloth bathrobe—the only clothing I didn't feel was cutting off my oxygen supply—and sit on the floor near my coffee table, which doubled as a giant-sized TV tray.

Beginning the ritual I was far too familiar with, I'd turn on the TV and start the food fest, cramming as much as I could down my throat until I was so sick I could no longer focus on the television. At that point I'd move into the bedroom, lie on my bed, and stare at the ceiling until the pain went away.

The pain from bingeing was intense. I could feel the food topping out of my stomach around the bottom of my throat, and from inside my chest I felt a terrible burning sensation that nothing would assuage—not water, not deep breathing, not even economy-sized Alka-Seltzer. I would have buckled over from this self-inflicted pain on a daily basis had it not been for the fact that buckling over would have caused the pain to intensify.

After the initial pain passed, I'd eat more. I'd eat as much as I could. And then I'd place whatever leftovers into the garbage and take it outside to the dumpster, usually late at night so none of the neighbors would see me. I didn't want the temptation of having the food in the apartment, even in the trash, during the night. I was always convinced that, somehow, the next day I was going to get the motivation to stay on a diet of some kind.

But that motivation never materialized.

I always *tried* to start anew. No matter what diet it was. And there were always plenty of new diets to try. And boy, did I continue to try them all.

Dr. Atkins, Scarsdale, The Beverly Hills Diet—you name it. I was especially fond of the crazy diets that were featured in many women's magazines: The Rice Diet, The Cabbage Soup Diet, The Eat-Anything-You-Want-Of-One-Thing Diet, etc.

At the same time I was also making up my own diets—usually consisting of three meals a day of "diet" frozen dinners or some kind of diet drink accompanied by diet pills—you name the brand, I tried most of them.

What I didn't know is that many of those frozen dinners were filled with enough sodium to send my blood pressure skyrocketing, which at over 450 pounds, I'm sure it was already doing even though I was barely into my twenties.

And I stayed on the diets, too. Usually until 5:00 p.m. That's about the time my willpower would give out, and I would either head to the grocery store or order in from restaurants that delivered.

Oh, how my mood would swing upward dramatically once I decided I would cheat. I mean, sure, I hated the idea of cheating, but somehow I knew *this time* would be different. This time would be the last time. And that thought, combined with the imminent binge, created a mental high like no other. The illusion of hope can be so intoxicating.

After I picked up my food order or had it delivered, I'd be very optimistic about whatever diet I was going to be trying the next morning. If I was at the grocery store, chances were I was buying binge food for that night and diet food for the next day.

It was a sick, sick cycle. Yet it was during those moments right before I took the first bite of my binge food that I was at my happiest.

All seemed right with the world. *Momentarily.*

But it wasn't right. I had become a recluse and basically lived in a fantasy world. When I wasn't watching movie rentals or TV shows, I was creating my own worlds through my writing. I would imagine elaborate scenarios and set pieces. Action and adventure was a favorite theme of mine—stories in which unlikely heroes would save the day. But even though I was committing these ideas to paper and writing movie scripts, I never shared them or sent them to anyone.

Contact with my parents had dwindled down to virtually nonexistent. One of the few times I heard from my father during that time was when he called to let me know that he had cleaned out some storage and had a bunch of Lori's and my baby pictures, along with a box of old family photos that he no longer wanted. It seemed having them around bothered Bonnie.

The armor I had surrounded myself with—humor and nonchalance about pretty much everything—always cracked whenever I had to interact with either one of my parents. I was hurt by Dad's callous announcement that he had no need to hold on to any of those photographs, and I was even more insulted when he asked me if he should just "throw them away." I immediately protested and asked him to mail them to me. He said if I wanted the photographs I would have to drive down to pick them up. He and Bonnie were still living in Florida at the time.

When I arrived at my dad's place, the icy apathy I was greeted with chilled my bones and broke my heart. Clearly Dad's feelings or rather lack of feelings for his only son had not changed. My baby sister Nicole was the only family member who showed any human emotions toward me. I picked up the box of pictures and brought them back to Tallahassee, where I placed them in a photo album for posterity's sake. Those memories may not have been important to my dad, but they were precious to me.

Thanks to the old photographs, I was now a little more in touch with my past, but I was virtually ignoring my present. I wasn't returning phone calls or writing to out-of-town friends. I wasn't seeing local friends. I would only use the phone to call my friend Kathi-Jo, who lived in New Orleans. She had moved there after college to be near Charlie, the love of her life.

Kathi-Jo and I were carrying on a clandestine relationship, as Charlie had "forbidden" her to communicate with me. The reason? He was convinced I had been trying to break them up while we were all in college together. I'm pretty sure this was because Kathi-Jo and I would have long conversations (which included lots of laughter) that Charlie could never quite wrap his head around. How could we possibly be having so much fun talking about nothing? This would result in late night phone calls, early morning phone calls, skipping class together, and more. So I guess I can understand why Charlie might have thought I had an agenda of erasing him from Kathi-Jo's life. But nothing could have been further from the truth. But even so, Kathi-Jo was too in love with Charlie to risk telling him that she and I remained friends.

Still, Kathi-Jo's and my long-distance phone friendship managed to flourish, and because of that we were convinced we single-handedly contributed to the rise of the phone company's profits as long-distance calls were still billed by the minute at the time. Our monthly phone bills were astronomical.

By being a shut-in I was missing out on every opportunity to lead a healthier lifestyle. I was never outdoors, I was never active (hence getting out of breath just from talking on the phone), and I never had any reason to try to look presentable.

It was a vicious cycle from which I saw no escape.

One fateful day my friend, Tasha, arrived at my door and started pounding on it. Initially I gave in to my usual shame and avoidance and pretended not to be home—but my car in the apartment complex parking lot had given me away.

Tasha continued to knock until I finally let her in. She stormed into the living room and demanded I get dressed immediately. Then she made her edict: She was going to the movies and I was going with her.

I protested. I complained. I gave excuses. But Tasha wasn't going to take no for an answer. We ended up going to the movies.

The experience was quite unsettling. Just getting out of the car at the movie theater parking lot took every ounce of courage I had. And this was despite being with my usual social "shield"—a strikingly beautiful woman. Up until now, if I was seen out in public with someone I deemed model-worthy, I had been okay to venture out. But I had grown to loathe myself and my appearance so much that even with Tasha I was afraid to be seen by anyone else. I felt like the "beast" to her "beauty."

I don't remember what movie we went to see. What I do remember is being squeezed into the movie theater seat next to Tasha, my fat spilling over onto the shared armrest, hoping she wouldn't notice my labored breathing.

Surprisingly, I survived. Tasha and I made it through the movie, back into the parking lot and back home where I was safe at last.

I couldn't believe it. I had made it into the outside world for something other than buying food. People had seen me in the light of day. And while it was uncomfortable, I lived to tell the tale. To this day I am grateful for Tasha's intervention.

I had finally reentered society. So when my friend Kathi-Jo encouraged me to visit her in New Orleans, I did. Only it turned out to be a big mistake. Upon arriving at her tiny apartment, I saw the shock and horror on her face. I was larger than she remembered. I had continued to grow after she had moved away from Tallahassee.

Throughout my stay, Kathi-Jo would come up with different reasons why she didn't want me to come out with her and meet her friends. Finally I called her out on her behavior. I accused her of being too embarrassed to have a friend the size of a house and that she didn't want to be judged by her new friends for having a friend that was so enormous.

Kathi denied it, saying she was still new to the area and just wasn't that social yet. But in my heart I felt like I was mostly being confined to "visit" her in her apartment. We barely ventured out on the town at all.

Prior to my New Orleans visit, I had experienced the prejudice of strangers on the street. But now I felt like I was experiencing that prejudice from one of the people closest to me.

Around the same time, I was beginning to notice that my friend Elizabeth would affectionately touch everyone she talked to—usually a pat on the back, a touch on the leg or hand, and so on. But Elizabeth never touched me, one of her supposedly closest friends.

Did I have some disease she was afraid of catching?

For the first time in my life I found that my anger, this time directed at Elizabeth, benefited me. Despite my insecurities, I began making it a point to join Elizabeth on her social occasions in order to prove to the world that fat people won't inflict any kind of disease on anyone else.

SMELLS LIKE MEAN SPIRIT

I was becoming a very defensive and mean-spirited person, full of bitterness both toward myself and others. Convinced that everyone in the room was making fun of my weight, I began to pick out their flaws and make fun of them to Elizabeth or whomever I happened to be with.

No one was safe from my caustic remarks. I gleefully poured my acid on the young, the old, the attractive, the not-so-attractive—they were all targets of my insecurity, shame, and years of bottled-up pain that lived within the layers of my fat. Because I believed I was *their* target. Sometimes I was. Sometimes I wasn't. And sometimes people couldn't have cared less about me. My self-centeredness took form in my inferiority. And my anger grew and grew . . . and I *raged*.

About that time I discovered something that overweight comic Louie Anderson had always joked about to be very true indeed. Mr. Anderson had a bit that talked about how thin people are always wondering if overweight people know they're fat. And you know what? He was right—people *do* wonder.

I noticed that whenever I brought up the word "diet," "blubber," or any fat-related-speak, people's mouths would drop open. It was as if I were a murderer confessing my sins. To my surprise, once those sins were confessed, I was forgiven—especially if I confessed and then somehow worked my obesity into a joke.

Suddenly I had discovered the wonderful world of "humorously" cutting myself down. I'd sit at a table and immediately begin the assault of jokes that ended with me or my girth as the punch line. I had people laughing in the aisles. Or in their seats at the very least.

But I wasn't content to let it rest with a few jokes with friends or strangers. I was ready to show the world that I had poundage to be proud of—and to laugh at. Okay, so I wasn't really proud of it. But somehow I think I was trying to come to terms with the blubber— and perhaps to acknowledge its existence to myself for the first time in my life.

I was now working part-time for a singing telegram company (Singing Tallygram—as in Tallahassee, Florida). I was answering phones, helping with the books, and taking phone orders. It was the perfect gig because I was able to wear my one pair of sweats and alternating nightshirts to work as I never had to deal with the public directly.

I had an excellent working relationship with my boss, Donna Smithey, who also happened to be the owner. One day, I approached her with an idea.

Donna's business thrived on sexy male ("Officer Friendly") and sexy female ("The Playboy Hunny") dancers. I suggested that we develop a novelty "sexy" male dancer—someone who weighed over

450 pounds. Someone who could maintain the necessary dance beat while taking it all off. Someone who would go for laughs instead of lust. Someone like . . . *me*.

Donna was open to the idea, and admitted that she had come up with the same idea for a Singing Tallygram act but wasn't completely comfortable approaching me about it. She gave me some ideas and direction, then told me to work up the act and audition for her just like all her other dancers had to do.

So I worked. I toiled. And then one fateful afternoon I introduced Donna to my brand-new act, The Mucho-Macho Gram (as named by Donna).

The act started off with me entering the room, wearing sloppy sweats and eating from a large bag of potato chips—then singing "Happy Birthday" (or somehow marking whatever occasion was being celebrated by the recipient) and acting depressed the entire time. I would then rope the recipient into asking me why I hated my Singing Tallygram job and then proceed to tell her that it was because I wanted to be a sexy dancer and that just because I'm big boned, I should still have a chance—that I had the "right stuff."

At that point I'd get very excited and ask if I could try out my new act that I was secretly developing. I then threw down the chips and hit play on my handy portable boom box. The theme song from *Flashdance*, *What a Feeling*, as sung by Irene Cara, would begin to play as I danced and writhed to similar moves that Jennifer Beals and her dance double made famous in the 1983 film.

Flashdance was followed by Klymaxx's *Man Size Love* during which I'd strip down to a T-shirt and tighty whities. (Yes, *really*.)

Donna loved my act and was willing to add it to her repertoire, as long as I was truly comfortable performing it. Since I'd be paid $25 for less than a half hour's work, I was comfortable. And so began the life of Tallahassee's newest stripping sensation.

The act quickly became very popular. I found myself performing at office parties, in restaurants—even at sorority houses—all in an effort to make people laugh at my tremendous size. You see, to me, the laughter was acceptance. People were no longer avoiding me like I had a disease. They were laughing. Some with me, some at me. But they were acknowledging my existence, nonetheless.

So at last, now that I was working as a stripper, life was almost acceptable because I finally felt like I was in on the joke.

However, in the meantime . . .

A funny thing happens when you apply to graduate school half-heartedly: You don't get accepted. And that's exactly what happened to me, which forced me, after a year, to admit defeat and move to Fort Leavenworth (near Kansas City) to live with my mom and her new husband, Joe, an army captain.

Joe was a nice enough guy. He went out of his way to make me feel welcome in their home, as long as I realized that their dog, Bear, a beautiful Irish setter, came first.

Bear had the run of the house. And if you don't believe me, I can show you years and years of their family Christmas letters that go on and on about Bear's antics, then mention Joe's son from his previous marriage and then mention—wait . . . those are the only "kids" mentioned in those holiday update letters.

One day while snooping around—an activity inspired since childhood by me wanting to know what my mom was up to "behind the scenes"—I found my mom's will. She left everything to Joe. Should he be dead, everything went to Joe's son, who was living with Joe's ex-wife in Texas at the time. There was no mention in Mom's will of me or Lori.

Matters were made worse one evening when I was talking to Joe out on the patio. Desperate to feel a little affinity, I made a concentrated effort to get close to Joe, thinking it might somehow get me accepted into this "family."

I opened up to Joe, sharing my concerns about being overweight and my fear of being fat for the rest of my life. To my surprise, Joe was very compassionate. And then he said, "Well, normal fat people deserve the shame, because they can do something about it. But your mom explained to me that it's because of a medical condition that you're fat."

Come again?

Apparently Mommy dearest was so embarrassed by my excess weight that she had concocted a lie about some disease I supposedly had in order to explain my size. I was incensed by Joe's comment. *How dare he?* No one deserves to be the victim of prejudice no matter what the reason for the condition they're in. I was infuriated.

But I hadn't even started feeling truly angry until Joe told me that I should be happy my mom went to the trouble of researching my medical information after my adoption.

My what? (Not again!)

Joe went on to insinuate that Lori was also adopted. So I guess after a brief tenure during which my mom claimed Lori as her own, it was back to both of us being adopted.

After this latest "you're adopted" confrontation I was left a little confused. I ended up calling my dad and asking him point blank if Lori or I were actually adopted. I'd felt I needed to, even though I really did already know the answer. My dad told me, "No," and confirmed that he and my mom were our natural parents. Strangely, he didn't seem that concerned about *why* I felt compelled to ask such a question.

And no, Dad's confirmation did little to quell my angst over this matter.

I finally realized that no matter how long I wished, how long I hoped, how long I fought, my mom was never going to change. She was quite content living in her fantasy world of lies.

Apparently she had Joe believing she was a French princess whose family lost their fortune and sent her to the United States. It was all so comical and pathetic at the same time. Comical unless you had the misfortune of *actually* being related to her. For Lori and me it was as if we were living a real-life nightmare.

I needed to find a job immediately so I could afford to move out of my mom and Joe's house and give their dog, the "only child" status he deserved and to get as far away as possible from my mom's web of lies and deceit.

Trying to find a job in the Kansas City area was a nightmare. After achieving more than decent college grades and ending up with many recommendations from a number of my professors, I had a strong presentation on paper. Every day I'd assault the help wanted ads and send out applications along with my resume— including every reason why someone should hire me. The initial responses were incredible. It was time to go on job interviews. Thus began my foray into the wonderful world of oversized clothing for business people.

I found myself surrounded by racks and racks of loud, Hawaiian-style shirts and easily stretchable polyester pants. Was this some kind of punishment for being overweight in the first place? Why some designer decided that overweight people don't deserve attractive clothes is beyond me. Buying pants with a size sixty-inch waist is punishment enough. Never mind having to buy them in the ugliest shade of gray you've ever seen. But buy them I did. I had no choice. I had in-person interviews to go on with potential employers who were very impressed with my resume and phone skills. I held down the phone's mute button when my breathing began to get labored so they wouldn't think I was trying to have phone sex with them.

I was dressed and ready for my first big job interview. My "business best" may have more closely resembled a circus tent than a working professional's regular attire, but I was dressed nonetheless.

My very first interview was for the manager position at a new gaming arena in Overland Park, Kansas. The manager was excited to have received my resume. In fact, he called me on a Sunday and asked if I could come in that same day, telling me I was all but hired and that he had even already checked my references. I was thrilled. At last I was "fitting" into the real world.

Arriving at the yet-to-open arena, I knocked on the glass doors at the main entrance and waited for the manager to arrive. Once he did he would not open the glass doors. Instead, he talked through the glass asking what I wanted. Putting on a brave smile, I explained who I was, reminding him that I was the guy who practically had the job.

He couldn't hide the shock as his eyes grew into large round orbs. Either he had just witnessed me murdering a small kitten or I weighed over 450 pounds. Since I had never tortured any small pets or any animals, I assumed it was my weight. Something this person didn't seem likely to get past.

He grudgingly opened the doors and showed me back to his office. After taking a seat I had a two-minute interview. Literally two minutes. He did all the talking while avoiding any eye contact whatsoever. Then he said he had several more interviews lined up and would be in touch.

Needless to say, I never heard from him again.

And so the process continued. I'd often get as many replies as the number of resumes I sent out. The only problem? I'd eventually have to meet these interested parties in person. And when they saw that I weighed as much as I did, their eyes would fill with fear, disgust, or horror.

Here I was, a bright, young college graduate, experiencing the kind of prejudice that would make people shudder. Often the interviewer would never look at me directly after the initial shock of seeing me. As with the gaming arena manager, there would be no direct eye contact whatsoever. Instead, they'd ask me a few questions and then send me on my way. For the most part, they were merely trying to go through with the interview in order to avoid being accused of any prejudice.

There were many times I wished I had filed some kind of complaint—not for my own sake—but for the sake of overweight people who followed in my footsteps. But I never did. The shame of my girth silenced me.

It's sad how easily society tolerates prejudice against overweight people. It's bad enough that we're forced to confront a "thin, gorgeous world" while trying to find underwear in our size, but to be at the mercy of someone who's decided we're less of a person because we're too much of a person is insane. And it hurts like hell.

After months of searching the help wanted ads and suffering through soul-crushing interviews, I finally succeeded in snaring two offers.

Interestingly enough, one was with an African American-owned company that managed several McDonald's fast food franchises. It was from this organization, that for obvious reasons encouraged ethnic hires, that I was offered a job because they saw me for *who* I was, not *what* I was. I was pleased with their job offer, but couldn't imagine working so close to all those McDonald's burgers day after day.

The other offer—and the one I ultimately accepted—came from a company headed by a woman who also happened to have a weight problem.

Cathy was a scream—the kind of brassy, balls-to-the-wall manager who would remind people that "We all put on our bra one strap at a time." She also saw me for who I was and immediately related to my life residing in "fat hell."

Once hired, I was able to take my cat and move into my own apartment in trendy Overland Park, Kansas—away from Mom, Joe, and Bear, the dog. I longed to become like the young attractive go-getter types I was writing about in my secret screenplays. If they could be wildly successful after their college years, then so could I. In other words, I was once again comparing myself to unrealistic media images, only this time ones I'd come up with myself.

In my bachelor pad I set up a stylish interior, complete with a guestroom for whenever company would visit and that doubled as a home office for writing the movie scripts I still wasn't telling anyone about. I began my daily drudgery of nine-to-five. For the record, it was more like 8:30 a.m. to 9:00 p.m., including some Saturdays.

The job with Cathy had me working at a proprietary college that specialized in "degrees" so that people could get jobs as medical and dental technicians. The kind of school you see advertised on daytime television. I was running the college's telemarketing department, where it turns out lots of overweight people worked.

Once again society felt like it was okay to stick overweight people in a crowded room in the back of a building where none of the general public would have to experience our girth. After all, over the phone we sounded just as normal as the next guy, right? Still, it was an avenue for employment, and I soon was making friends with coworkers who worked in other parts of the college.

Cathy and her husband became good friends of mine. Since they were also overweight, we could all relate to the feeling of being at the opposite end of society's attractiveness scale. They helped me integrate myself into the Kansas City social scene and always made me feel welcome. We'd often go out drinking or eating after work and frequently did something silly to boot. Gluttony seemed to be something all three of us had in common.

One time we all ended up crowded inside a small, filthy video booth in an adult bookstore, daring each other to put a quarter in the slot to get our video peep show. How the three of us fit into that small booth is beyond me, but I guess it goes to show where there's a will, there's a way.

While an adult bookstore wasn't the normal place to be doing so, hanging out with Cathy and Gary made me feel like "This must be what it's like to have a good relationship with your parents." They had children of their own, but they showered a lot of love and attention on me. And it felt really good.

GOING CLUBBING

As my social life picked up, so did my desire to trim down. I was getting sick of wearing sixty-inch waist pants and even squeezing into those on most days.

There was a well-appointed health club, the Athletic Club of Overland Park, located near my apartment complex that I investigated courtesy of their one-week free trial membership. I was a nervous wreck, but I managed to find some oversized workout wear and forced myself to go on the sixth night of my free trial membership.

This club had a reputation for being the place where the "beautiful people" worked out. As much as I wasn't one of the "beautiful people," I knew that I wanted to be friends with them.

Working out there was scary. I was surrounded by spandex-wearing gods and goddesses with curves in all the right places. To make matters worse, the club's walls were mirrored, giving me a "four corners view" of my wide-load body. I had trouble doing things with the same agility everyone else seemed to possess as they accomplished their exercise routines.

Surprisingly, no one yelled at me, and no one seemed to be horrified at my presence, so I decided to join the club. I began by walking around the indoor running track. My goal was to be doing brisk walking, but reaching that modest target took a little while. Shortly after meeting that goal, I decided that I was ready for my first aerobics class via baptism by fire. I owned several home exercise videos—many of which were still wrapped in plastic—but I felt there was no real way for me to "practice" aerobics without getting into the actual classroom.

Attending regular aerobics-style classes was intimidating. Once again I was in a mirrored room, surrounded by what seemed to be the cast of a modern version of *The Stepford Wives*. There I was, hot, sweaty, and obese, sure I would start an earthquake when I was stomping to the beat of the latest "High NRG" music. But I survived.

I even managed to win over my aerobics instructor. It wasn't from my perfect aerobic techniques or graceful moves. I did it by bringing her little gifts every Friday night, kind of like a pupil bringing his teacher an apple. Regardless of my methods, I soon became a respected member of the club.

I learned a lot while attending that club. I had the good fortune of befriending the club's athletic director, Steve, who also happened to be a sports nutritionist. Steve was very compassionate and took the time to teach me some of the tools I would need in order to finally begin to tame my blubbery beast.

I didn't realize it at the time, but I was acquiring several helpful hints that would eventually come together years later and help me conquer my inner demon.

There was just one hitch undermining my newfound workouts. After exercising, I'd make sure that I'd hit the drive-through window of some fast food joint on the way home. I didn't care about the extra mileage or, apparently, the extra poundage.

But as I became more familiar with some of the members of the club, i.e., the "beautiful people," and grew ever jealous of their trim, sleek physiques, I decided to get serious about my efforts, which ended the fast food follies and contributed to my joining Weight Watchers.

I had read a lot about Weight Watchers over the years and had even subscribed to their magazine. Still, the magazine alone didn't seem to help (perhaps because, although subscribing to it, I rarely read it). So I waddled into a local meeting one fateful day. Scared. Alone. Frightened.

The agenda was simple: join (by giving money), get your menu-plans, weigh yourself (at the scale in front of the Weigher), and then join other members by attending and supposedly participating in a one-hour classroom-type meeting, which was led by instructors who were reported to be former Weight Watchers members themselves.

I paid. I got my program book. Simple enough. My nervousness got worse when I went to get weighed. The Weigher was stunned when the scale didn't go as high as my weight did and shouted for her supervisor, not knowing what to do.

There I was, standing on the scale, a long line of people waiting to get weighed-in behind me. I was mortified. My fear and loathing only intensified when the Weigher re-entered with her boss, who also couldn't figure out how to make the scale go higher.

Finally Bea, the sprightly instructor for the evening, entered and attached a small thingamajig to the scale, which allowed it to register my weight. I didn't like what I saw, but I was grateful the ordeal was over.

Convinced that *this* was going to mark a new era in my quest to release the weight, I kept a journal of all my measurements.

GREGG'S WEIGHT WATCHERS MEASUREMENTS	
Weight	457.5 pounds
Waist	65 inches
Tummy	65.5 inches
Chest	56 inches
Neck	18 inches
Bicep	18 inches
Forearm	12 inches
Thigh	35.5 inches
Calf	19.8 inches

Bea turned out to be a pistol. She was a tiny little lady who one couldn't imagine ever having been overweight in her life. But she had been, and she spoke like she knew what she was talking about.

So I sat. I listened. I even took notes in the spiral bound notebook I brought from home for good measure. I was determined to make this work.

Bea was a wonderful instructor. She was often cautioned by visiting militia members of the Weight Watchers headquarters that she spent too much time veering off the planned lectures. It was true; Bea did often veer off. But it was because she wanted us to know all of the information she could possibly offer in order to help us win the battle of the bulge.

I think Bea could tell I was a special case. Upon meeting me, she introduced me to one of her favorite members of the group, Petra Allen. The first thing I noticed about Petra was her big, welcoming smile—along with her subversive humor. Here was a happily married Kansas City mom who was only too happy to buck the system in regard to what it meant to be a "proper" Midwestern homemaker.

Petra loved theater, was a talented writer and performer, and had a mom who was a professional actress and a husband, Bob, and son, Morgan, who were equally intriguing and welcoming of having me as a new friend. Petra had a bumper sticker on her car that read "Sundae Driver" and featured a charming illustration of a little pig driving a convertible with a giant sundae in the backseat. When I saw that bumper sticker I knew I'd met a kindred spirit.

Little did I know at that time that meeting Bea and Petra would be the highlights of that particular Tuesday night Overland Park Weight Watchers group. But at the start of this attempt, I was determined to make the dieting aspect of the program work for me—no matter what.

This time I was going to lose the weight—once and for all.

As many of you know, the dieting plans from Weight Watchers and similar organizations are based on food exchange groups that have been broken up into different categories: bread, protein, fat, fruit, and vegetable.

A typical day would look something like this:

Gregg's Typical Weight Watchers Menu

BREAKFAST

1 cup of Cereal

1 Banana

1 cup of Skim Milk

LUNCH

1 Peanut Butter & Jelly Sandwich

5 Potato Chips

1 Tangerine

DINNER

1 cup of Garden Vegetable Soup

1 small Broiled Pork Chop

1 small Red Potato

2 teaspoons of Reduced Calorie Margarine

SNACK

1 cup of Fruit Cocktail

1 cup of Skim Milk

All well and good—in theory.

But if your heart and soul aren't in it, it's amazing just how much "one tablespoon of peanut butter" can be. Despite all the meetings, all the handouts, all the talk, Weight Watchers never really helped me get in touch with *why* I might want to lose weight. Only *how*.

Still, the scale was kind . . . at first.

TALLIED RESULTS FROM GREGG'S WEIGHT WATCHERS BOOKLET	
Week One	Lost 12.5 pounds
Week Two	Lost 7 pounds
Week Three	Lost 1 pound
Week Four	Lost 2 pounds
Week Five	Lost 1 pound
Week Six	Gained 2 pounds
Week Seven	Gained 4 pounds
Week Eight	Gained 3 pounds
Week Nine	Lost 3 pounds
Week Ten	Gained 7 pounds
You get the picture.	

What was happening? All my initial success was dwindling as I headed back up toward 457.5 pounds. And here I had been "perfect" on the diet. Well, except for that one time. And, oh yeah, that other time, too. And . . .

Uh-oh.

My and many other Weight Watchers members' patterns were rearing their ugly heads. Sure, I was dieting. But I was also cheating. And that's because I was continuing the "on-and-off" mentality that wrecks almost every dieting effort.

Yes, I was losing weight. But I was *also* gaining it back because I was teaching myself how to cheat. Like other members of Weight Watchers, I was learning that by weighing in once a week, I could cheat for a couple of days after the weigh-in.

The only problem was that the cheating days would increase and soon they'd take over most of the week. The Weight Watcher who didn't experience that phenomenon was the exception, not the rule. And members all knew it, and we bonded because of it.

My new Weight Watchers pal Petra and I became members of a tight-knit group that attended the Tuesday night Weight Watchers meeting in our area. It was a well-known fact that after the meeting, we'd all go out to dinner and eat like pigs. This fulfilled a social need I had been longing for, but it negated the purpose of *why* we were getting together in the first place—to lose weight!

Week after week we'd pick a different dining spot, so that each member of our group could give in to his or her taste buds. It was ridiculous. Whether we lost or gained, you could find us pigging out afterward—and sometimes the next day, and often the day after that.

It was like members of Alcoholics Anonymous going out binge drinking right after a meeting. Where else are you going to find such enthusiastic drinking partners? The same was true for the food lovers enrolled in that particular Weight Watchers group.

While I gained some close friends through those meetings, and even a lifelong friend in Petra, I also gained some close allies in cheating. We were like kids attending boarding school, ignoring the teacher until the bell rang and then heading off to the trough.

The folks at that Weight Watchers group would always be very forgiving of a weekly gain. Why? Because they wanted me to come back the week after that. Why? Because they wanted my money the week after that.

A typical exchange went something like:

WEIGHT WATCHERS WEIGHER: "Weight gain? No problem. You'll try harder this week!"
ME: "Yeah, yeah—sure. Give me my booklet so I can go."

There were many weeks that my Weight Watchers friends and I would meet prior to the meeting, weigh-in, and then take off for the restaurant, skipping the evening's lecture altogether.

In sixteen weeks I had barely lost twenty-six pounds total. Now, added all together, I'd lost over sixty-two pounds. But I'd also gained several pounds in the interim. Up and down. Round and round.

Even though I continued to yo-yo up and down the scale, week after week, I thought Weight Watchers was my only hope. I decided to turn the other cheek and ignored my crazy yo-yoing, determined to believe I was finally conquering my weight problem. Yet deep down, I longed for something more.

NO TELL MOTEL

I now had a fairly active social life with my friends from work and friends from Weight Watchers, but I was still lonely. People enjoyed being with me, but it was rare that they wanted to touch me—even in the form of simple pats on the back or friendly hugs. And when it came to other forms of intimacy, well . . . those were nonexistent. There was never any potential of romance waiting to happen in my life. Much less a friend or two who would pat me on the back like they did other, thinner people. I felt like a leper.

And so it happened that one night I drove to a Motel 6 located on the side of a remote highway about twenty miles from my apartment. Once I checked in, I looked in the motel room's Yellow Pages to find and call an escort service.

I was ashamed and embarrassed, but I needed to be touched. I needed to feel loved, even if I was going to pay $200 for it.

When the escort arrived, I could barely make eye contact. It was all very business-like. The money was to come up-front. It would last just an hour, even though all I wanted was to be hugged.

That's right. No sex. Just intimacy. The kind that comes from feeling someone warm next to you, with their arms around you, unafraid of the "obesity disease" that the rest of the world seemed to fear.

Perhaps Weight Watchers could have arranged "hugging night" so that those of us who needed to know we were still human could be assured of just that.

I spent two month's worth of spending money in one night, simply to have someone hug me while I watched a local newscast silently play out on the motel's television set in the far corner of the room.

Afterward, I sat there on the edge of the bed feeling my flesh grow cool where the escort had held me. I tried to hold on to that warmth and the belief that I was part of the human race, but instead the whole experience made me feel more alone than ever before.

ANOTHER PERSPECTIVE
ON GREGG AT THIS TIME

By Donna Smithey, Gregg's Singing Tallygram Boss

Reading these pages, I'm struck by the differences in how one person perceives another and/or the events taking place in their lives. My perception of Gregg while he was in Tallahassee was completely different from what he has described here.

Of course, at the beginning of my long friendship with Gregg, I did notice his weight. But after that initial observation I moved on to focus on the person inside. My relationship with Gregg was filled with humor, happiness, fun, and great respect. He was a person who would accomplish anything he set out to do. I remember he was constantly shooting horror films around town. These student films weren't bad either. At one point he sent a music video clip to an MTV music video contest and was one of the top contenders. He seemed to excel at anything he tried.

Once he arranged a "Hollywood Premiere" for one of his student films at a local downtown cinema. He wrote, directed, and edited the film. He handled all the marketing, took care of the details and made it happen. I never felt so proud as when I walked up to that theater and saw lines of people the length of a city block waiting to get in. What an accomplishment! I knew at that point he would be successful at whatever he set his sights on—regardless of his outward appearance.

Gregg helped me tremendously with my first business in Tallahassee—The Singing Tallygram Company. We were always looking for something different to put out there, and so the Mucho Macho Gram was born. He and I had so much fun creating that routine. I remember both of us falling on the floor laughing. Any suggestion I gave, Gregg was all for it. I asked over and over, "Are you okay doing this in public?" He assured me he was. You have to be a very secure person on the inside to turn an outward appearance into a funny character out in public. This turned out to be one of the best characters (besides the Nerd, which hadn't been developed yet) attributed to Singing Tallygram. To this day, people still approach me about both Singing Tallygram characters.

Gregg also helped me on my weekly radio show, *Show Talk*. This was a one-hour show that covered arts and entertainment for the northern Florida area—I had opened two community theaters in Miami, worked at the Asolo Repertory Theater, and received a masters degree in Theater from FSU—all pre-Gregg McBride. The show had many special artistic guests, both local and national, when they were in town for the FSU School of Theatre. Regardless of who the guest was, Gregg made sure to call in to keep the phone lines from going dead with "callers" who wanted to ask the guests questions. He had different sounding voices he used when calling in, so as to sound like different callers during the same show. He was a true original.

I knew Gregg worried about his weight, but I also knew that a person has to be ready to deal with a serious issue before they can be successful in conquering it. I knew the time would come. It was painful for me to read these pages and realize what a dark place Gregg was in during our time together. I knew there were ongoing issues but not to this extent. Yet I saw success written all over him—no matter which path he chose. I saw him as a kind, fun, and giving person. And yes, I experienced the brown bathrobe. It did not give me nightmares or send me running to analysis.

I also saw Gregg as very social person. He had my niece and me over for Thanksgiving one year, at his apartment that he sometimes hid away in. The place was lovely. The food was scrumptious and he couldn't have been more attentive and giving. I still remember that Thanksgiving fondly. His weight never bothered me. I loved being in his company. He made me feel very special, which I imagine he does with every one of his friends to this day.

ANOTHER PERSPECTIVE
ON GREGG AT THIS TIME

By Petra Allen, Gregg's Weight Watchers Buddy

I had forgotten that it was Bea who introduced the two of us, though I have no doubt Gregg and I still would have found each other very quickly at those Tuesday night meetings.

Gregg had that instant charm and wit, an easy laugh, and a ready smile that totally belied the angst that filled his soul. Only later did I learn about this and begin to understand the extent of his self-consciousness. I also can't remember when I realized Gregg only liked to gather "attractive people" around him—his enrollment at the Overland Park Athletic Club being a strong indicator.

My own self-consciousness would never have allowed me to consider such a thing! I was close to my ideal weight and knew how to dress and how to apply make-up stylishly, so I felt attractive enough for Gregg to accept me into his world. I saw his world as one of infinite possibilities due to his intelligence and creative spirit. Not for one minute did I doubt his ability to lose weight and achieve any goal he set for himself. I saw the "essence" of Gregg, which outweighed any extra weight his body was holding onto. I saw his soul and he saw mine, whether we realized it from the beginning or not.

We had the weight loss in common, of course—plus we shared a passion for the theater and performing. We also shared a love of laughter and a finely tuned sense of the absurd, but likely it was the capacity for pain in our spirit that bonded us most. We talked to each other, we listened to each other, we encouraged each other, and we accepted each other. Unconditionally. It was (and is) what any good relationship should be. For me, meeting Gregg equaled finding a kindred spirit, someone who "got me" and whom I also understood and could advise from having lived life years longer and having a solid, loving, and open relationship with a spouse and child.

I didn't see the extreme neediness in Gregg. It was my husband who saw that and expressed his concern, pointing out that Gregg did not need me to be his mother. That comment came after a Saturday morning visit from Gregg, where he was sitting at our kitchen table, needing my attention due to some heartfelt issue when I should have been more engaged with my family.

Perhaps we were the family Gregg had always yearned for and wanted to be a part of. I never saw that as a problem. Maybe Gregg did depend on me more than would be considered healthy, but what harm was done? Possibly I filled a void that Gregg carried in him for years. Isn't it a wonderful thing to be a balm for an aching soul?

My family was not neglected as a result of my friendship with Gregg. To this day he includes my family in all his greetings and correspondence. Plus, I too benefited from our friendship by having someone to laugh and cry with over our weight loss foibles and our weekly "cheat dinners" after weigh-ins. A lot of laughter went on during those dinners. I don't think they were counterproductive, because the social bonding and acceptance was worth so much!

Ultimately, Weight Watchers was the right thing for me, and I learned how to have a healthy relationship with food, including indulging in that occasional splurge. I enjoy my free monthly visits to a meeting as a lifetime member. Most importantly, I will forever be grateful to the organization for the lifetime friend I found there in Gregg.

CHAPTER FIVE

i'll eat manhattan

I was nearing my mid-twenties when I decided that I'd never have real love, at least not while weighing as much as I did. And at that point, I was pretty sure I was going to weigh at least that much for the rest of my life.

Sure, my now predictable Weight Watchers dieting and bingeing cycle had somehow helped me take off around fifty pounds, but I was still overeating regularly in order to fill my insides with what was missing:

No career. No love. No hope.

Well . . . maybe a little hope.

No longer satisfied with being hidden away in the college's telemarketing department, my thoughts were turning to more fulfilling career dreams. Specifically, my dreams were of being a filmmaker where, for once, my weight didn't seem to be such a terrible thing. Some of history's most successful filmmakers also happened to be some of the *largest* filmmakers around. Thank you, Alfred Hitchcock, Orson Welles, and Rob Reiner.

I had been secretly writing scripts for years, but was never willing to show them to anyone aside from the two student films I wrote and directed while attending FSU. I finally decided it was time to share my new scripts with others.

I set my sights on Third World Newsreel's Advanced Film Production Workshop in New York City, an annual program for college graduates who hoped to get into the entertainment industry. After filling out the extensive questionnaire with lengthy essay questions and submitting a writing sample, I learned I'd been selected for the in-person interviewing process.

I flew to Manhattan—the pride of New York State—glamorous, exciting, and vibrant with life, and went to the workshop location only to find out that it wasn't held in the more upscale part of town. As a matter of fact, it was in one of Manhattan's least glamorous locales: Hell's Kitchen. That area of the city has since been "cleaned up," but at the time it was known for its high crime rate.

This was a huge change for someone who went to college in Tallahassee, Florida, and spent his first year as an adult in Kansas City, aka "The Heartland," but I was willing to make the effort if this earnest group of filmmakers was ready to take a chance on me. And they were.

As it turned out, I was the minority in the group. Not because of my weight—though I was the only morbidly obese student—but because of my skin color. Third World Newsreel was a program set up for students of color who might not otherwise be able to study film. Once again, a rare occurrence: People were seeing me for who I was and what I offered, rather than for how much I weighed and how I appeared on the outside. I was lucky—and honored—to be accepted into the program.

Taking evening classes in Hell's Kitchen took a lot of adjusting to. I would take the bus from New Jersey, where I was staying with my college friend Elizabeth while I was looking for my own place, into Manhattan's dreadful Port Authority, New York's bus terminal, more aptly described as hell on earth with the smell of urine permeating every crevice.

As I walked to class, I'd keep my hand in my pocket, my fingers strategically positioned around the contraband can of Mace I'd tote into the city for safety's sake. After class, I'd once again hold tight to the Mace and walk back to the bus terminal, praying I wouldn't end up as a featured victim on *America's Most Wanted*.

Often, once I was safely on the bus, I'd realize that I had my hand in the wrong pocket with my fingers tightly placed around a canister of Binaca breath spray. In other words, I'd been on the verge of giving muggers fresh breath and then spraying Mace into my own mouth. Thus began my adventures in New York City.

Despite my many failed attempts, I was still trying to diet. After all, with constant dieting, I had a reason to constantly cheat. The Northeast coast of the United States introduced me to a whole new variety of foods to indulge in.

My favorite feasts while living in northern New Jersey and studying film in nearby New York City consisted of hitting a local Montclair, New Jersey deli where I'd order up at least three Italian submarine sandwiches at one time. We're talking fat, fat, and more fat, all tucked between a fatty bun.

Could you add a little extra oil and mayonnaise on that?

I supported myself and my intensive eating habits with two jobs. One, working as a sales person at a local gift shop, The Cat's Pyjamas, and another as a waiter at a local franchise restaurant, Houlihan's.

Getting both positions while weighing so much was definitely a triumph and both made for some very interesting encounters.

Gail Ingalls, the owner of Cat's Pyjamas, was a woman who later confided in me that she was sure she wasn't going to hire a man for her store a second time. Past experience had taught her not to do it again, because men were usually not creative types and couldn't sell the inventive novelties she featured in her shop and national catalog. Imagine her surprise when she hired not just any man, but a

400-plus pound one, someone who would need to squeeze behind the different display cases located close to the store's walls.

Before the interview, I had been warned by a local resident that Gail prided herself on being the area's trendiest owner of the trendiest shop. That terrified me. Flashbacks of the "beautiful people" came flooding into my mind. I thought of myself as a fairly trendy guy; I was an aspiring filmmaker who tried to keep his hand on the pulse of whatever was considered "current." But I also weighed over 400 pounds, and had to make do with the most un-trendy wardrobe options from the local Big and Tall Stores.

Putting on my Sunday best I headed off to the interview, complete with a lump in my throat. Upon meeting Gail in person, I saw her reputation was accurate. She was a beautiful woman who dressed the part of one of Manhattan's elite.

Gail didn't blink twice when she met me. She didn't seem to be concerned at all about my girth. The only thing that concerned her was my schedule—and my willingness to work nights and weekends. After less than half an hour, I was hired. Boy, was I surprised. Didn't she know society classified me as a fat pig—an un-trendy fat pig at that? Apparently not. Gail was willing to take a chance, and I'm thankful to her to this day.

Working for Gail worked out beautifully. Yes, there were some tight-fitting spaces behind those jewelry counters, but somehow I managed. What I lacked in mobility, I made up for in character. I treated the small, trendy boutique as if it were a major department store—sending customers to "Gift wrap on floor seven" (the next counter over) or answering the phone with cheerful greetings: "Santa's Helpers shop at Cat's Pyjamas." I had customers—and Gail—laughing constantly. That proved to be good for business, which was good for me.

One of Gail's full-time employees was a sassy girl named Sally Gentile. With her jet-black hair and pale white skin Sally was what you'd call a New York club girl—dedicated to the latest trends and usually discovering them a couple of years ahead of the rest of us—and not an easy nut to crack. Sally not only worked in the store, she also did all the business's bookkeeping and was thus privy to Gail's inside scoop. She made it a point not to fraternize with the part-time help.

What Sally didn't realize was that I was going to make her laugh. And laugh. And laugh. I also created music mixes for the store, the variety of which impressed Sally. She had me pegged for "all pop, all the time," but I showed how eclectic my musical tastes were and that she shouldn't judge a book by his cover.

Getting hired at Houlihan's Restaurant was a longer, much more grueling process. It was basically a repeat of my unpleasant experiences in Kansas City, only this time with a happy ending.

For those of you not familiar with Houlihan's, you might know it as Bennigan's, T. G. I. Friday's, or any number of chain restaurants that are more than a Denny's but less than a four-star dining spot. It was a generic "good times" place with overly decorated walls, offering dishes that could choke the arteries of the healthiest athlete.

I was called in for an interview by Bill, the manager on duty, who, after hearing about my experience and seeing my resume, told me over the phone that I was "practically hired." When I introduced myself in person I could tell Bill was stunned by the sight of me and my weight. In fact, he must have been so put off that he couldn't even talk to me. He promptly passed me off to his assistant manager, Kim.

Cute and thin, Kim spent the entire interview staring down at my resume and doing all the talking. Then she thanked me for coming in and told me there were currently no positions available. I guess they had filled them all during the hour since they had initially called me.

I was used to that kind of treatment, so I continued working at The Cat's Pyjamas. But one day I got a call from Peggy, another manager at Houlihan's. Apparently Kim had neglected to throw out my resume, and to inform Peggy, the latest manager, that they didn't need any new servers. Peggy called me in and did something that anyone on a job interview would appreciate—she looked into my eyes and got to know the real me.

I started at Houlihan's immediately afterward and became a star player on the wait staff, much to the dismay of Bill, the first manager, and Kim, the cute, thin one—who were open-mouthed when they saw me at the next server orientation. ("Hi, guys!" I enthusiastically shouted out when they saw me. *Oh, yeah . . . I went there!*)

Despite my girth, which was admittedly something to contend with when rushing through the crowded restaurant, I worked to become the branch's star server. This included being the waiter of choice for several restaurant regulars who I was told had connections to organized crime. In other words, everything about their dining experience needed to be *perfect*. This was never a problem for me. Often I would approach a table of guests and see the shock or disgust in their eyes when they saw my size. That's when I'd make sure my service was first-rate and came with a healthy dose of my sense of humor in order to turn their opinions around. Most of the time my strategy worked. Soon the mob-connected patrons were asking for me by name, and I don't mind telling you they were big tippers.

During this time I applied to various medical insurance companies at the urging of my father. Ironically, insurance companies wanted nothing to do with the obese. I was unable to get insurance due to my weight. Never mind that I could have lied on the application form, but I refused to do that. The fact that I was attending Weight Watchers meetings in an effort to lose the excess weight and was very active on my feet at the restaurant didn't seem to matter.

I finished the film program in New York City, and was left with both of my part-time jobs. While they were fun, and while I had friends, it was time for something more. Yet a career in film didn't seem to be happening at that time. The thought of moving to Los Angeles and *really* going for what I wanted to do in life was just too frightening. What if it didn't work out? What if they hated fat people even more in Hollywood than they did in the rest of the country?

The uncertainty was too much to bear. So I stuffed those movie business dreams down with my next three submarine sandwiches.

It was time to think about full-time work here in the Northeast part of the country. And I found it through connections at the restaurant, landing a copywriter position for Macy's Department Store's advertising department. That's right—working right there at the site of *Miracle on 34th Street. Heck,* I thought to myself, *If I'm not going to use my creative ability for Hollywood, I'll use it for the advertising industry.*

I was hired by a woman who happened to have a soft spot for The Cat's Pyjamas' catalogs.

Working for Macy's was fun. It was exciting. And it was terrifying. Because without realizing it, I had entered the high-end fashion industry. At the time, Macy's was still known for setting and creating trends with all the best designers—before the eventual bankruptcy turned them into the Mecca of all sales emporiums.

My department was staffed by a bunch of young, cute, thin artists and writers. I was young. But that was it. I had trouble fitting into the tiny cubicle, let alone relating to all the buying trends my new coworkers were constantly talking about.

Jean Paul Gaultier and Donna Karan were not designing clothes for those of us wearing "larger than average" sizes. I was still relegated to the wonderful world of king-sized clothing. I will humbly point out that I had the finest footwear around, however. I may not have been able to wear Ralph Lauren Polo around my waist, but I could wear it on my feet.

Convinced that an overweight person was never going to fit in, I was still desperate and made every attempt to do so. It took a while for the trendy New Yorkers who populated the advertising staff to accept me into their clique. Not surprisingly, there were some who never did. But others eventually embraced me.

One such embracer was Karen, a tall, beautiful Nordic blonde, who garnered positive attention from anyone who encountered her. I was proud to be seen with her about town on lunch breaks and such. And surprise! Karen loved to eat as much as I did. So it was that we bonded over the three o'clock coffee breaks that always involved one of us running downstairs to get snacks from the local kiosk. To be clear, Karen actually *ran*—I took the elevator.

On special days, Karen and I would abandon our cubicles and trot down to the store itself, which populated floors one through eight, and visit the Cellar or Epicurean Shops where we could delight our taste buds with not only delicious, but expensive, foods.

I was still on Weight Watchers. On Mondays. And sometimes on Tuesdays. By Wednesday (the morning after weigh-ins) I was on my own eating plan.

Gregg's Typical New York City Diet

BREAKFAST

1 large Fat-Free Muffin with Carob Chips

1 small carton of 2% Reduced Fat Milk

2 Bananas

MORNING SNACK

1 Candy Bar

1 cup of Coffee with Heavy Cream

LUNCH

2 Ham and Cheese Sandwiches

2 small bags of Potato Chips

2 Hostess Cup Cakes

2 Diet Cokes

AFTERNOON COFFEE BREAK

2 Hostess Twinkies

2 Candy Bars

1 cup of Coffee with Heavy Cream

1 Diet Coke

DINNER

1 medium-sized Steak

1 Baked Potato with Melted Cheese

Broccoli with Melted Butter

3 pieces of Cake

3–4 Diet Cokes

NIGHTLY SNACK

1 Apple

Gee . . . why wasn't I losing weight?

THE WRITE STUFF

I thought I was as happy as could be, even though I was basically ignoring my exercise and dieting programs. However, I noticed that I wasn't being invited to certain meetings at work—meetings for the Juniors, Jewelry, Swimwear, Infants, and Kids departments within Macy's (all areas of the store that my writing duties were supposedly meant to cover).

I eventually realized it was the advertising department's vice president, Alan, who didn't feel like I fit in or belonged in the meetings. I asked Karen if my suspicions were true and she begrudgingly admitted they were. I believed Karen, because while she was tall, blonde, and beautiful, she, too, was battling a smaller-scaled battle of the bulge.

I guess that after I confided in Karen, she decided to take me under her wing. She was a hotshot art director for the department and began to demand that I was the writer assigned to her many, often high profile, projects. The department had no choice but to listen, and soon I was attending the previously forbidden meetings. I think this shocked my boss, Joan, more than Alan, the VP.

Alan noticed that just because I wasn't picture perfect by the fashion world's standards, I still had a lot to offer. In fact, I often had insights that these buyers had never thought of before. Soon enough, I was seeing my campaign slogans not only in the huge display windows on 34th Street, but also in national fashion magazines—and it was thrilling to say the least.

Meanwhile, my boss Joan, who was a writer herself, seemed to be angry that I was somehow outshining her, a fact I never wanted to believe was true. It's interesting how some people's reactions to you change once you break through whatever barriers they had set for you in their own minds. I guess Joan had intended for me to write the sales ads ("50% *off*" or "Save 50% *on*") and never imagined I'd advance to loftier ad writing duties.

Fortunately, I didn't spend a lot of time worrying about Joan. Instead, thanks to Karen's dedication and my writing abilities, I became the toast of the department. There I was, yes overweight, but always invited to the most important meetings and the most fashionable modeling agency parties.

The agency parties were the hottest tickets in Manhattan. To be invited meant you were one of New York's elite, or at least you could pretend you were for the duration of the party. They were populated by supermodels, agents, actors, and musicians. And having your name on "the list" and being ushered in through the VIP entrance was pretty heady stuff for this guy who was formerly known as "foxy for a fat kid." The music was always loud and up-to-the-minute, the drinks were always free, and each event boasted a hip, frenetic energy that can be experienced nowhere else except in The Big Apple.

An invitation not only meant you were deemed "cool" by the fashion world, but that you would be allowed to party with the actual supermodels themselves and be able to partake of their open cocktail bars, as well.

More excess gluttony? I was all for it.

Looking back, I see that I used to make an idiot of myself at these parties. As soon as I was in the door, I would drink down as many of the free drinks as I could.

Why? The reason was simple. I was literally the *only* person in the club or whichever venue said party was being held at who was even the slightest bit overweight. I was surrounded by other people in the industry, most of them thin, gorgeous models. Even people who worked behind the scenes were model-thin and pretty darn attractive in their own right.

It was the entire "thin person in the catalogs"-"beautiful people" dilemma right there in my face. At one such party I sauntered up to the bar to order my first drink of the evening. Karen (my so-called protection and link to the "beautiful people") had dashed off to the bathroom, leaving me all alone at the bar. I looked up and found myself standing next to model-turned-actor Antonio Sabato, Jr.

In the mirror behind the bar I could see myself standing next to him. It was like a living, breathing "before and after" picture. To clarify, I was the "before" and he was the "after." *Way after.* I was horrified.

I drank my drink and proceeded to drink Karen's drink. Then I ordered two more and did the same thing again. I got pretty drunk that night—so drunk that when I saw a model who I thought to be Claudia Schiffer, I hustled over to her and asked her for a kiss. The alcohol had lessened my inhibitions, but it also took away most of my self-control. Ever obliging, the beautiful creature leaned forward and planted a small kiss right on my lips.

"Are you Claudia Schiffer?" I asked.

"No," she answered with a thick accent while shaking her petite blond head.

This striking young lady was named Berta and she was just starting out in her modeling career after arriving here from the old country. No matter. There was a smoking hot beauty willing to kiss the fat, horrible beast.

I dashed off into the dark club to gather up my friends from Macy's in order to have them witness this budding romance. Once the crew was gathered, Berta somehow saw fit to give me another peck. I was in heaven.

My public rendezvous with Berta was as close to romance as I was going to get. Though I had once been chased down the street by an admirer who was a self-professed "chubby chaser," I knew a real romantic relationship was not to be had for me. Not unless I wanted to pay for it again, which I did not. I wanted all of my extra income to go toward food.

There I was, surrounded by thin, gorgeous, glamorous people, people I longed to be even further integrated with. I had to do something about my dieting efforts. One thing I found out about most of the models I was meeting was that they were always willing to share their tips on staying thin, as long as you asked. Since I always felt compelled to let them know I *knew* I was fat, I always *did* ask. But not all of them kept their svelte figures through healthy living. Some of what you hear is true; many models depend on seriously scary crash diets as a means of keeping their photogenic selves looking good.

It was about that time when I dropped out of Weight Watchers. I wanted to lose weight the fastest, quickest way possible. And that common sense dieting menu wasn't going to do it.

This began my plunge into the scary world of crash diets—an approach that has been known to result in the death of those who become too consumed by them.

I freely admit that I *tried* to become bulimic. It seemed to be the supermodels' diet of choice. So one night, after I pigged out on as much Italian food as my stomach could handle, I went into my bathroom and stuck a finger down my throat.

No reaction.

I then grabbed a toothbrush and stuck that down my throat.

Nothing.

I then grabbed a hair brush and shoved the handle as deep into my throat as I could. My eyes watered as I gagged at the feeling of the large handle making its way into my mouth. I coughed. I hacked. But still I didn't get the desired reaction.

Apparently my body was not about to give up even one slice of the large pizza I had just consumed. I realize now how lucky I was that my body didn't respond to that unhealthy practice.

Bulimia is a terrible battle to fight, and one that would have been very seductive for someone like me. At the time I was very upset that I couldn't be more like the bulimic, skinny models I knew.

So instead I decided to double up on the diet pills. My thought-pattern went like this: If one pill was good, then two pills were better. Needless to say I got little sleep during that phase of my life. Ironically, there were many late nights when I would head out and buy food just because I couldn't sleep.

Charlene Piro was a thin, sassy friend of Karen's who worked as a traffic coordinator for our advertising department at Macy's. She was young, hip, and beautiful, always dressed in black and perfectly svelte. That's right, I hated her. And I always felt like she hated me and probably was wondering why Karen ever befriended me.

Then one day, while strolling through our aisle of cubicles, Charlene stopped by to go a few rounds with me. By "rounds" I mean trade a few sarcastic jabs. I was able to keep up with her thanks to my wit; okay, thanks to my bitterness. After my final zinger, she smiled at me in her signature way, half grin, half wince and said, "I like you."

Apparently Karen had told Charlene about my sense of humor and Charlene wanted to investigate it herself. I was flattered. Charlene could have been a character on the classic TV show, Sex and the City. Only she would have eaten the rest of the lead characters for breakfast.

I was never that comfortable around Charlene, always sure that she was about to lower the boom and drop pig's blood on me (a la Stephen King's Carrie). I couldn't believe someone I deemed "this cool" actually wanted to spend time with me, without some ulterior motive.

The crash diets and diet pills and attempted bulimia weren't helping my self-esteem any more than Charlene's sincere admiration was. The more I tried the crazy, dangerous diets, the heavier I became. I found myself less active and I got more sickly. All of a sudden I was over 450 pounds again.

How could I tell? Because along with running out of breath while talking on the phone, my knees hurt more and my heart was constantly racing. I was straining to fasten my sixty-inch belt around my waist. Even sixty inches were becoming too few for my rotund midsection.

I decided to go back to that "healthy-minded" diet, Weight Watchers. Once again I was a gerbil running on an endless hamster wheel. For a while there were a few weeks during which I would take off up to seven pounds. But then I'd also have weeks during which I would gain back just as much.

There were no friendly Beas at those East Coast meetings. In the New York metropolitan area, Weight Watchers was a massive machine where we dieters were to be rounded up and shuffled through like cattle. Apparently they were even shuffling through their very own Weight Watchers instructors, since many of them were as heavy as the students. Yet they continued to proclaim their diet worked.

Sure their diet worked, that is if you didn't cheat and reported to all of their classes. But that was something I wasn't able to commit to . . . *ever*.

I was so frustrated. My dieting and bingeing cycle was spiraling out of control. I would lose and gain thirty or more pounds within the same month. I tried desperately to talk with many of the Weight Watchers instructors, all of whom told me to "Just hang in there."

One fateful night I attended a meeting with my pal Elizabeth in tow. I held my Weight Watchers booklet, in which they register your weekly weight, in hand as I stepped onto the scale while the cold-hearted Weigher had to once again fumble around for the necessary attachment in order to weigh me.

Once she figured out how to use the scale, we both saw that I had gained fourteen pounds in one week. *Fourteen* pounds! Can you imagine?

I burst into a cold sweat and told the Weigher that I needed help. She handed me my freshly tallied Weight Watchers booklet and said, "That's why you're here. To get help. *Next*."

That was it. My Weight Watchers breaking point.

I turned around to face Elizabeth and told her I was no longer going to participate in Weight Watchers' "bandage on the dam" approach to weight loss. I was sick of it. Having seen me go up and down the scales over and over again, poor Elizabeth didn't know how to respond.

The night was still young, so I dragged Elizabeth to the nearest Friendly's restaurant where I proceeded to eat more in one sitting than I ever thought imaginable.

Gregg's Quitting-Weight-Watcher's-Binge

1 Double Bacon Cheeseburger

1 Fried Steak Sandwich with Extra Mayonnaise

1 large order of French Fries

1 large order of Onion Rings

1 large Reese's Peanut Butter Cup Sundae

1 extra large Hot Fudge Sundae

1 Root Beer Float

4 Diet Cokes

Elizabeth just sat there with me as I ate and while other people in the restaurant stared in amazement at me pigging out. I was the only one eating at our table. It was nighttime and Elizabeth was just having tea.

I was like a helium balloon filling up to the brink of popping. I didn't stop eating until I was, literally, about to burst. Elizabeth didn't know what to say or do. She knew what I was doing was hardly the cure for what I called my Weight Watchers blues.

There's nothing Elizabeth could have said that night. All I wanted to do was eat until I was no longer thinking about the scale and, instead, only about how much pain I was in. Little did I know how close I was to ending the mental and physical pain of being obese once and for all.

ANOTHER PERSPECTIVE
ON GREGG AT THIS TIME

By Sally Gentile, Gregg's Coworker at The Cat's Pyjamas

When Gail, my boss at the time, told me she hired Gregg to work in the store, it was big news. Not because Gregg was "big," but because she had actually hired a man to work in the store. Until then, Gail had never had any luck finding men who had the right kind of personality to sell pink plastic flamingos and other novelty items to the well-to-do housewives of Upper Montclair, New Jersey. But Gregg, she said, had what it takes.

"Oh, and by the way," Gail added, "He's really big."

So I have to admit Gregg's being big was also somewhat surprising. Not because I thought Gail held any prejudice against larger people, but because I knew that the space between our display cases and the walls was pretty tight. Not even Gail, who was waif thin, could do a 180-degree turn without hitting a wall. But Gail felt Gregg had enough command of his body to handle the tight spaces. And as it turns out, he did.

As the company's bookkeeper, I didn't work in the store that often, mostly just during the busy holiday rush. So I never made it a habit to get to know the part-time help well, also because they came and went pretty quickly. But Gregg had a spark and a sense of humor that I couldn't resist. He and I became good friends and would often hang out and go out to eat together.

At the time I was living at home with my parents to save money, which meant that whenever Gregg called or dropped by to pick me up, my old-school father would put him through the paces—as if Gregg were a fifteen-year-old boy coming to pick up fifteen-year-old me. It was hilarious, and Gregg handled my parents just fine. He even ended up using them as on-camera talent in a TV commercial for a local bakery that he wrote and directed. He always knew how to win people over. Because of that I never thought much about his having difficulty in life due to his size.

The topic did come up from time to time, although it was mostly when Gregg started to lose the weight. Some of our mutual friends began treating Gregg a little differently, as though his losing weight somehow intimidated them. One woman we both knew well even encouraged Gregg to cheat. It was as if he no longer fit into the "perfect friendship puzzle" she had constructed for herself. It wasn't surprising Gregg stepped away from that friendship soon after. He was determined to reach his goal and I applaud him for that.

Gregg was never one to complain, and so he didn't talk much about his issues with his mom. I do remember picking him up at the airport one time, when he was returning from visiting her and her then current husband, Joe. Gregg got in the car and just started crying. He couldn't tell me why he was crying. He just sobbed. I leaned over, patted his knee and told him to "Just let it out." And he did. I had never seen Gregg cry before, and I haven't seen him cry since. His tears were so heavy I can't help but remember that tough moment for him.

We've been friends for a very long time now. I always thought "through thick and thin" was a random saying, but when it comes to my friendship with Gregg, the phrase definitely applies—and, in our case, also literally.

CHAPTER SIX

ready for takeoff

The irony of a 450-plus pound man working in the fashion industry was not lost on me. While I thought I was fitting in for the most part, that really wasn't the case. Thanks to Karen, the art director, Charlene, the traffic coordinator, and Alan, the vice president, I had earned some acceptance within the department itself. But I still hadn't accepted myself.

Once again I was clocking in at a weight that had me squeezing into my largest-sized clothes, holding my hand over the phone speaker so people wouldn't hear how winded I was just from a phone conversation, and sneak-eating high calorie snacks anytime someone wasn't looking. I would even throw used candy wrappers away in other people's trash cans so the janitors at the office wouldn't be aware of my binge cycles.

Still, there was no hiding what had become my daily morning struggle to wrap my sixty-inch belt around my waist and get it to buckle using the last available belt hole. The strain on the belt was showing via loose threads and worn leather. The Big and Tall stores closest to where I lived didn't sell any sizes above a sixty-inch waist. Soon I was going to have to place special orders for clothes that would fit me. Something had to be done.

I wasn't sure where to turn—or *who to pay*—for the next "cure."

I don't know if I'm embarrassed to admit it was vanity that drove me to look for a winning strategy to conquer my battle of the bulge once and for all or if I'm proud of that fact. Arguably I should have been more motivated by my rapid heartbeat, pained knee joints, and breathless phone conversations than by thinking about how I looked. But I was working in the world of high fashion, and aside from the occasional "pity kiss" from a kindhearted fashion model, I clearly wasn't *fitting* into my surroundings.

So I set my sights on someone who *was* fitting in. I figured if I had a role model of sorts, I could zero in on what exactly it was going to take to beat this challenge and once again be able to buckle my belt without reciting a "Hail Mary." After all, I wasn't even Catholic, much to the chagrin of my fifth grade girlfriend, Ann.

This is when I began to take notice of our department's vice president, Alan, a little more closely. He was thin, handsome, athletic, funny, happily married, and a parent to adorable kids. Add to that his successful career in fashion and you had my new go-to guy in terms of someone to idolize or, rather, someone I hoped to *emulate*.

I had caught Alan's ear in regard to the advertising copy I was writing for magazine fashion ads, but we weren't very close. Plus, I didn't feel comfortable talking to another man about my weight issues. Most members of the weight loss groups I'd belonged to over the years were women. Yet I felt I had to *man up* and approach Alan. He seemed to have everything I was looking for.

But how? How did he have it? How did he get it? And where did I need to sign up for the same?

In my mind Alan was privy to some sort of secret to "having it all." I figured if I played my cards right and asked him at just the right moment, he might actually share that secret with me.

One day after a copy meeting, I saw Alan alone in his office. I decided this was the moment. No one else was around. I would make my move and let him know I had a weight problem.

I marched into his office, shut the door, approached his desk, cleared my throat, and waited for him to look up at me. After a moment, he did. This is when I announced, "Alan, you may or may not have noticed that I have a weight problem."

Insert long pause here. *As if* he didn't know I had a weight problem. I was around 450 pounds, after all.

Alan blinked and then stared at me blankly. Not knowing what to do next, I began to ramble.

I told Alan about my childhood. About my abusive parents. About all the things that plagued me and *forced* me to start eating and gain weight. If only I had already written the previous chapters of this book, I could have just handed them to him to read.

Alan's stare continued. I was nervous; I was anxious. I couldn't stop wondering what incredible secret this thin, athletic man who apparently had everything and was able to *eat* anything and stay trim was going to offer to me. And then, his lips suddenly parted. He prepared to speak. Bright white light seemed to shine down from the heavens! I could hear angels begin to sing! I *knew* I was about to be handed the key to the universe from this insightful, sagacious creature.

Alan's words?

Alan's secret?

Alan's key to living a life of being thin, fit, and happy?

"Just stop eating so much!" He said glibly.

Huh? No, wait . . . I wanted real advice, man. This is what I was thinking to myself instead of saying it out loud. Although I'm sure my gaping jaw communicated the same thing. "Is there anything else?"

Um . . . No.

I thanked Alan, then quickly retreated from his office, invisible tail between my legs, moving down the longer-than-it-ever-seemed-before hallway, back into the heart of the advertising department and to the safety of my cubicle where a drawer full of candy bars awaited me to start eating so that my shame could be digested.

Alan might not have shown me compassion, but there were three Musketeers who were willing to.

As I secretly administered my chocolate first aid, I decided I wasn't going to waste any more time with someone like Alan. Someone who clearly didn't understand the anguish, the pain, and the prejudice I had gone through and still was going through in my life. I knew in my heart that all of my trauma added up to some very real evils that were conspiring to keep me fat against my will.

In other words, I knew that *none of this was my fault.*

Later, I shared Alan's callous remark with a few heavy girlfriends. Like me, they found his response rude, insensitive, and crass. They agreed with me. I agreed with them. Then we all finished the ice cream sundaes we were cheating on our diets with.

Days went by. The food intake continued. There was no way for me to weigh myself at home since my electronic scale would only register ERR. It was official. I was once again the size of a small country.

But as my massive intake of food continued on a daily basis, so did my obsession with what Alan had said to me. *Just stop eating so much!* It made no sense. It had no value. No *weight.*

I would see Alan on occasion, living his life, eating anything he wanted to, fitting into his clothes with ease, enjoying lots of friends, introducing his beautiful wife when she would drop by the office. He knew the secret to losing weight and looking great, and yet he hadn't been willing to tell me what that *real* secret was.

When I pointed this out to my friend and coworker Charlene, she told me she thought his advice was "Right on."

I should have known Charlene would say that. After all, she was thin and beautiful herself. Sure, she was always complaining about five pounds she wanted to lose, but her sexy figure, tousled hair, and *au courant* wardrobe told me that she was also privy to Alan's secret. And like him, she wasn't willing to share it with the resident fat guy in the department.

I decided I didn't need Alan's or Charlene's top secret information. Instead, I would just secretly observe them when they weren't looking—watching what they ate, spying on their interactions, taking note of how they were living their lives. I was convinced I would be able to decipher all of the ways in which they "secretly" stayed thin and beautiful.

After much observing and note taking, I didn't come up with what I thought was helpful information on how to transform my life. If I had paid more attention at the time, I might have picked up on their food choices, their portion sizes, and their nonlethargic ways of moving around the office. But because of my "fat thinking," there I was, once again back at "square one."

Just stop eating so much? *As if.*

I was also once again spending the weekend only with myself and my thoughts. It was late on a Saturday night and all sorts of crazy notions raced through my mind. It was almost as if my inner demons were trying to confuse me now that I felt like I was starting to break through the clutter of years and years of mixed messages in regard to what it would take to get healthy.

I took a gallon of ice cream, emptied it into a large plastic bowl, covered it with Oreo cookies and then squirted chocolate syrup over it—my idea of a light snack before bed. I sat down on the couch, turned on the TV, and started to eat.

Saturday Night Live was just coming on, and actor and comedian John Goodman was the guest host.

As I pounded down the ice cream, I could feel my heartbeat beginning to race and my breath beginning to quicken, the usual side effects of binge-eating. I didn't care. I wanted to be thinking about my heart racing and my breath quickening, *whatever,* to keep my mind off Alan's nonsensical "just stop eating so much!" advice.

At that precise moment I noticed the side effects of being obese demonstrated by John Goodman on television. He was just standing on stage, doing the monologue at the top of the show, but he was sweating profusely. And he was completely out of breath. All from just standing there, talking.

I couldn't believe it. This amazingly talented performer looked as if he was about to collapse. This is when I realized I wasn't looking at John Goodman on TV as much as I was looking into a virtual mirror at *myself*.

My mouth clamped down so hard around my spoon that I remember hurting my teeth on its cold metal surface. Suddenly, I was acutely self-aware. Time and my rapid heart beat seemed to stop for a moment. And in that moment . . . that very moment . . . when . . . everything . . . *changed*.

I looked down at the half-eaten bowl (barrel) of ice cream. I stood up, calmly walked into the kitchen, put the remaining ice cream and cookies down the drain, and turned on the garbage disposal. A little of the ice cream splashed up out of the drain, as if it were desperately calling for help, hoping I might reconsider what I was doing. But I kept the water running and the garbage disposal on until all evidence of the binge was gone.

Only this time, I wasn't hiding the evidence. I was declaring that a new day was dawning.

Alan's words now weren't confusing me as much as they were beginning to resonate within me. *Just. Stop. Eating. So. Much.*

Taking off the weight was simply about making an attitude switch—a *simple* life change. It wasn't going to take a lot of thought or a lot of therapy. Nothing like that. It was as simple as changing the channel from The Food Network to ESPN.

The following Monday, I put on a different kind of detective hat. I was going to research healthy eating. This meant checking out books at my local library, scanning nutrition-minded as opposed to *diet*-minded magazine articles, and even booking an appointment with a doctor recommended by Charlene who could help me outline the necessary ingredients for a healthy eating plan.

Key word: *Healthy* (eating).

Even though I weighed over 450 pounds, I wasn't investigating dieting as much as nutrition. I wanted to create a diet that would give me everything I needed to be healthy. No false humility here. I still wanted to be thin and stylish. But I wanted that to be a result of my lifestyle, not some crash diet. I had already tried all the crash diets. Usually more than just once.

The doctor let me know that portion control was something I needed to pay attention to whether I was consuming tomatoes or chocolate. He added that weight loss was mandatory immediately; otherwise, I was soon going to need some kind of joint surgery on my knees and/or other areas of my body that were starting to give out under the enormous strain of my excess weight.

The task of developing a healthy eating plan was overwhelming, but also thrilling and exciting. I could tell I was really onto something. And within a few weeks I was following my simple, self-made regimen.

A Typical Day on Gregg's New Diet

BREAKFAST
1 cup cooked Brown Rice, served warm, sprinkled with Cinnamon

½ cup of 2% Reduced Fat Milk

½ of a medium Banana, sliced into chunks and mixed into the Brown Rice

LUNCH
Lunch Salad

6 oz. of Skinless Sliced Turkey

2 cups Fresh Salad Greens (usually a mix of Lettuces)

Carrot Shavings (for added texture)

Dressing

Small mixture of Olive Oil, Balsamic Vinegar, and Dijon Mustard

DINNER

2 cups Chunky Turkey Chili (recipe shared on page 265)

Small Side Salad (Lettuce, Tomatoes, Cucumber)

Dressing

Small mixture of Olive Oil, Balsamic Vinegar, and Dijon Mustard

EVENING SNACK

1 to 2 cups of Fresh Fruit

AND THROUGHOUT THE DAY

Lots and lots of Water (room temperature)

For a treat, I'd have Sparkling Water with meals

I'm not going to lie to you, that diet initially sucked. I felt like all of the food I was eating tasted like cardboard. I learned that was because I was used to consuming nothing but junk food with countless additives and other artificial ingredients, which meant I didn't really know what *real* food tasted like.

Sure enough, within the first couple of days (even *hours*) of that diet, I decided I was going to cheat. There was just no way I could do this. It was torture, plain and simple. I decided cheating was going to happen during lunch on the first day of my new diet.

As I sat in my cubicle at Macy's, practically French kissing the plastic salad bowl in order to lap up every last drop of salad dressing leftover from the salad, I looked up. Alan walked by. He didn't say "Hi." He didn't even notice me. His stride was confident. His clothes looked comfortable. His attitude was in tow.

"Take a picture, it'll last longer," said a brassy voice from behind. I turned around to see Charlene, who wanted to know how the diet was going.

I shrugged my shoulders, knowing I was still planning on breaking said diet.

"Well, you look great. I can already tell you lost weight."

Of course, Charlene was just being encouraging since it was the first day and no real weight loss would have been visible yet. But her encouragement gave me the strength I needed to make it through the rest of the first day of my new way of being.

This was especially difficult around 3:00 p.m., when someone from our department would do the daily run to a downstairs food cart for afternoon coffee and snacks. I robotically put in my order, and then realized that I wasn't able to partake in this activity anymore. I felt crushed. I felt robbed. I felt like life was unfair.

But somehow I made it home to my dinner, then an evening snack, and finally, bedtime.

As I lay in my bed, cuddling with Shadow, it dawned on me that I had gotten through an entire day without "cheating." Sure, I thought about getting up out of bed and driving to the nearest fast food restaurant. But I was very tired. Exhausted in fact, because my body wasn't getting the usual amounts of caffeine and sugar it was used to. So I closed my eyes, deciding I would cheat the next day.

Yet, I did not cheat the next day, despite the enormous headache I had, not to mention the mounting depression. My whole way of analyzing my world seemed to be thrown off course. Charlene joked that I had all the same symptoms of her mother, who was going through menopause at the time.

Yeah, Charlene, that must be it.

SCALING BACK

Much to my amazement, I still hadn't gone off of my diet. I was approaching the two-week mark and I was desperate to know what I weighed. I still couldn't weigh myself at home.

I made an appointment with the doctor to weigh-in, as well as check-in. I was still committed to the health-minded aspect of all this, and not just the vanity aspect. The doctor was surprised to see me so soon, but willing to weigh me since he had a scale that could have attachments added to it in order to weigh someone over 400 pounds.

I stepped into the small room where the scale was and the doctor added two attachments to the scale—one so that the scale could register a weight over 400 pounds and the next for registering a weight over 450 pounds.

Now came the moment of truth.

The doctor told me to step onto the scale. *Clunk*. The scale register sank to one side. I began to panic.

"What's wrong?" I asked. "Do you need to add another attachment?"

I dreaded the answer, since if the scale did require that, it would mean I weighed over 500 pounds.

"Not exactly," said the doctor as he *removed* one of the attachments.

Suddenly, the scale balanced out. Turns out I weighed 435 pounds. I'd dropped over fifteen pounds in the first two weeks of my dieting efforts.

At 435 pounds, I felt as light as a helium balloon.

I wanted to grab the nearby nurse and kiss her, then break into a musical number. The doctor could tell I was giddy, and he was excited for me. But he cautioned me that a lot of this was water weight (*argh!*) and that the longer I stayed on my diet the more slowly the weight would come off. But he added that as long as it was coming off, *that* was the important thing.

Then he said something that really bummed me out. He wanted me to start exercising.

"Even with my knee joint issues?" I asked, reminding him of a reason why I should have permission to be lazy.

He replied he wanted me to start exercising right away since "Getting healthy requires a two-pronged approach." Diet *and* exercise (*sigh*). He gave me a stern look that had me quickly retreating from his office, still anxious to break into a musical number after taking off more than fifteen pounds of excess weight. I didn't care whether it was water-related weight or not!

Certainly I had lost a dramatic amount of excess weight close to that in the past. But I'd put it all back on again. Then I'd take off a little more. Then put on a little more—and so on. I knew that was my pattern. But this time I was determined to arrest that pattern. After "releasing" those latest fifteen pounds, calling it "release" rather than "loss" since I didn't want "loss" to insinuate I was giving up anything, I was determined to continue my dieting efforts.

I still wasn't really tasting the food I was eating, much less enjoying it. At that point the headaches and depression had subsided, but I still wasn't finding pleasure in the experience.

Looking back on that time, I see I was acting somewhat like a robot. I chalked up the reason I followed my doctor's orders and enrolled at my local Bally's Fitness to "robot mode." I hadn't thought about regular exercise in a long time. But doctor's orders were doctor's orders. And I was, thankfully, a robot.

I was lucky this gym offered late night aerobic classes, since working in New York City and living in New Jersey required a lengthy commute that didn't make me available for exercise until after 8:00 p.m.

When first showing up for aerobics, I was relieved to see the class was made up mostly of women. After years and years of weight loss groups, I was still more comfortable with the ladies than with men, who mostly populated the free weight area at the gym. Still, I was sure those women would turn and stare at the enormous man in the back of the mirrored aerobics studio. They didn't. In fact, I appeared to be somewhat invisible to them, which was fine by me.

I attended this evening aerobics class three times a week. And no, it wasn't easy. I was still running out of breath while talking on the phone, so you can imagine how breathless I got when shaking my groove-thing to the tunes of Janet Jackson and Mick Jagger, the instructor's favorite artists. But shake it I did. I was as robotically committed to the exercise as I was to the diet.

Along with being a robot, I felt like I somehow subconsciously became a racehorse with blinders on. I wasn't thinking about what was going on around me. I wasn't thinking of distractions. I wasn't focused on what I was giving up. I wasn't even really thinking about the finish line. Instead, I was simply thinking about moving forward in the moment. And forward is exactly the direction in which I moved.

As long as I would see downward movement on the scale, I was happy. Some weeks it was as much as seven pounds. Other weeks, it would be as little as half a pound. Still, I knew I was headed in the right direction. I remained committed to only weighing once a week and I didn't focus on one particular goal weight.

My doctor had advised that at 5′ 11″ (6′ if I stood up straight), a healthy weight would be around 185 pounds, and I was still too far away from that weight to realistically envision it. Instead, I would think in terms of fifty-pound increments as interim goals along the way. I was lucky that after my "first" weigh-in I had gotten below 450 pounds. So I next set my sights on getting under 400. Then I'd focus on getting under 350, and so on. To think of every pound I needed to lose to get to that elusive goal weight of 185 pounds was just too much to bear all at once.

After a lifetime of fast food addiction, preparing meals wasn't my favorite task. Especially with my long work schedule and now with an exercise schedule on top of that. I found that making food over the weekends and separating it into portion-friendly containers was the way to go. I was basically creating my own microwaveable meals—ones in which I controlled the ingredients.

I would often have the same meal daily. Yes, that meant monotony, but there was a certain comfort in doing things that way. After all, I was in weight-loss mode. And the weight was coming off.

So I developed a few favorite recipes that I still enjoy to this day. (See the Bonus section beginning on page 253.)

To my surprise, friends and associates at work were always very interested in what I was eating. Besides seeing me starting to slim down, they also said whatever I was warming up in the microwave smelled "incredible." A lot of times those smells would be wafting from my Turkey Chili recipe (page 265). Before too long, people were asking me to bring some for them, and eventually whenever I would be invited to a party, the hosts would request that I bring a big pot of the Turkey Chili to use as a dip. I was only too happy to do so, especially since it meant there would be something at the party that I could munch on without going off my diet.

Along with people clamoring for my Turkey Chili recipe, another great motivator was all the attention I was getting at work for my newfound "incredible shrinking man" status. People were amazed that I was *actually* losing weight this time—as opposed to just *talking* about losing weight, which I'd done incessantly up until then. Each week, right after I weighed in at the doctor's office, friends at work would take a Polaroid picture of me to chart the physical changes.

I think my coworkers were a bit awestruck by my success. I was still morbidly obese by society's standards, but increasingly less so than I'd been weeks and eventually months earlier.

Strangely, there were a few people who weren't quite sure how to deal with that "lesser" me. I suppose they were used to "fat, funny Gregg," and perhaps my changing in such a dramatic way took them out of their comfort zone.

My boss at Macy's, Joan, would often bring in cupcakes and other treats and leave them on my desk as a "surprise." At the time I didn't think much of it. But in hindsight her behavior seems like that of a saboteur. I would be very tempted but ultimately did not succumb to the seductive treats and gave them instead to Karen's boyfriend, John, a bodybuilder who was only too happy to gobble them up.

SOCIAL STUDIES

Partaking in my diet at work and at home was now rote. But social occasions still felt like dangerous waters. I'd been on my plan for a couple months and yet I'd never stepped foot in a restaurant of any kind. Restaurants were like Kryptonite to my Superman. I knew in my heart of hearts that I wasn't able to place a "special order" or anything of that nature. Yes, I know I *could have*, but I also knew I *wouldn't*. I knew that if I dined in a restaurant I would have instantly ordered the "fried so-and-so with sauce and a side of extra fat."

This restaurant ban became *de rigueur*, even if it meant missing out on a social occasion or two. In fact, social occasions themselves eventually proved to be just too mentally grueling for me.

Soon after I'd achieved some initial success, Easter Sunday was fast approaching. I was invited to Elizabeth's mother's house; home to a wonderful Italian woman who loved to cook and to see people eat what she'd prepared.

I decided that I would allow myself a "day off" from my diet. But somewhere deep inside, I felt that I needed permission to do so. I called my doctor and asked him what he thought about going off my plan "in honor of Easter Sunday." I was sure I'd couched my proposal in such an earnest manner that there was no way I would be denied.

"Nope," said my doctor bluntly.

"But it's Easter Sunday," I protested. "It's going to be really hard to stay on a diet on a holiday."

"Well, you just gotta do it," said the doctor even more callously.

I couldn't believe my doctor's rudeness. Didn't he understand what Easter was all about? It was about chocolate bunnies, jellybeans, and Peeps, not to mention Elizabeth's mom's authentic homemade pasta with homemade "gravy"—aka "spaghetti sauce" to us Italian wannabes.

But despite my internal protests, in the end I did not partake in Elizabeth's mother's Easter smörgåsbord. Instead, I brought my chicken lunch salad drizzled in un-Easter-esque Balsamic vinegar dressing and ate it in the corner while everyone else had the other goodies from the lavish buffet.

My resolve was soon tested again, this time at a picnic that Elizabeth held at the lake house she was currently staying in. I brought my friend Sally from The Cat's Pyjamas store as my date and we were both surprised by the enormous amount of food being served. Elizabeth had gone all out with the menu, which panicked both Sally and me, since she was also trying to take off a few pounds at the time.

Thinking ahead, I had brought my "lunch salad" with me which, surprisingly, put Elizabeth into a tailspin.

"This is a special occasion, Gregg," she said. "Not a day to be dieting." Her tone was terse. She was clearly very upset.

After she darted off to greet more guests, Sally and I took one look at each other and left the picnic. We decided our willpower wasn't strong enough to avoid the fatty salads and barbeque sauce-drenched meats. Instead, we snuck off to a matinee at a nearby movie theater. Elizabeth was furious with both of us and didn't speak to us for a long while as a result. But we didn't care. We'd stayed on our diets. And at the time, that's what mattered most.

After that picnic I decided social occasions were going to be out until I'd taken off enough weight to no longer be tempted or feel overly deprived. Not all of my friends understood that decision. And some may think that was the coward's way out. But for me it was a very brave commitment.

As the "fat kid," I longed for social occasions to validate me. But I made a choice of health over going out. A hard choice that ultimately led to my success. So for me, that was the necessary path. I knew that decision didn't have to be forever. But, just for that time period, it was what I needed to do to continue my momentum.

I decided, instead, to get to know myself a little better. After all, spending years with layers of blubber insulating me, which I used to put off *really* getting to know other people, had also kept me from really getting to know myself.

Why, I wondered, did I *want* to lose weight?

I bought a large, blank book, the kind found in bookstores and art supply stores, and used it to create a "success scrapbook" or what I called a Me Book. I would cut out words from magazine headlines that I found inspiring, articles about health and fitness that I found motivating, and pictures from catalogs featuring "thin people clothes" that I wanted to wear. I even put my "before" picture and my weekly weight into the book.

I basically kept my eye out for anything that I found inspiring— collecting ideas, articles, visual images, and other sources of printed inspiration that I would then glue into my scrapbook, which soon became my go-to bible for inspiration.

Anytime I was tempted to cheat or felt out of touch in regard to *why* I wanted to take off the excess weight, I picked up my Me Book and reconnected with the reasons why I *wanted* to lose weight. Yes, *wanted*. That "wanted" thing was something I would constantly have to remind myself of. Losing weight was a choice. And this time, I really *wanted* to do it. My Me Book helped remind me of this.

My Me Book became a real source of motivation for me. After all, I was on a journey. And chronicling that journey was not only therapeutic but also very inspirational.

Through my strict dieting efforts and three times a week aerobics classes, I was eventually able to weigh myself at home on my own scale, meaning I had finally gotten *under* 400 pounds and no longer needed to be weighed at the doctor's office. And the weight continued to melt away. Not as quickly as it did during the first weeks, but enough to keep me motivated. And the motivation only increased when the tracking of my success was made apparent not only by the scale, but by the strange occurrence I'd never really experienced before—*looser clothing*.

So this is what it's like to be able to breathe when wearing a belt, I thought to myself. The day came when the sixty-inch belt I'd been struggling to wrap around my waist needed to be replaced. That was a major achievement. I still have that sixty-inch belt and I treasure it as a memento to this day.

After several months on the diet, I not only had to ditch my belt, but also *all* of my pants. Sure, I'd bought a few pairs of "in progress" clothes at the Big and Tall stores along the way. A fifty-four inch waist might sound ginormous to some, but to me it was a sweet relief to pull those pants on after straining to fasten sixty-inch waist-sized pants for so long.

But there came a day when the fifty-four inch pants no longer fit. They were too loose. And so on. And so on. Until one day, I decided to step into a mystic place I'd often heard of, but had never actually been to. When going into a Gap store for the first time in my life, I decided to do it alone. Should things turn ugly in the dressing room, I didn't want anyone there to witness it. Not even one of my closest friends.

A friendly salesgirl greeted me with a smile. "Welcome to the Gap. What can I help you find today?"

I was sure she was being sarcastic. Surely she knew I belonged in the Casual Male Big and Tall store and had no business being at the Gap. I'm pretty sure my face was on a poster in the back of the store, warning employees not to let me in. But I quickly averted her stare, telling her I was "just looking." I must have done so in a convincing way because she turned her attention elsewhere as I darted to the back of the store where all of the men's jeans were.

I knew I had to work fast—before another employee or a security guard would approach me and escort me out of the store for being so obviously in the wrong place. I scanned the sizes, promptly locating the largest available: Size forty-two inch waist.

Looking in both directions to make sure the coast was clear, I grabbed a pair of straight-leg jeans and dashed to the dressing room. I took off my sweatpants and pulled these strangely sized jeans up over my thighs, around my waist and, low and behold, they not only fastened at the waist, but also zipped up!

I was breathless for a moment and began to lose consciousness. I snapped to as I heard what I was sure was the Hallelujah Chorus. No, Gap employees were not gathered outside of the dressing room singing, but I heard angelic voices in my head. That was a major achievement!

For the first time in my life I was wearing "average-sized clothes" for "average-sized people." I wanted to run out into the store and kiss the salesgirl. Instead, I looked confidently into the dressing room mirror.

I was experiencing a joy I had previously only gotten from eating. Only it was even greater now. At long last, I realized that what I'd heard over and over might actually be true: Nothing tastes as good as being thin feels.

Would this progress continue?

ANOTHER PERSPECTIVE
ON GREGG AT THIS TIME

By Charlene Piro, Gregg's Coworker at Macy's

I remember working in the advertising department at Macy's. I hated my job almost as much as my chain-smoking, authoritarian boss hated me. In the pseudo-fabulous fashion world of Macy's corporate advertising, I was caught between bi-level bob haircuts, big shoulders, out-of-control budgets, and crunching numbers. Nothing, it seemed, was going to make that job bearable.

And then one day, from across my cramped cubby, I saw a ray of happy hope coming to the advertising department—and it was emanating from someone who was almost as big as the sun itself. It was my future best friend, Gregg McBride.

Finally, a breath of a fresh-coworker, and he took up enough space for four of them.

My mind raced with a thousand thoughts: Where did he come from? How did he have enough time in a day to consume all those calories? Where did he buy those tasteful plus, plus, plus-size clothes?

Gregg was the kind of fat that caused heads to turn and whisper. Usually he kept those people laughing, perhaps with the hope that they would somehow overlook his layers of fat.

I am typically unfriendly at first, due to shyness. But Gregg brought out the best, not only in me, but in everyone around him. Perhaps he did that so as to combat his fear of not being accepted.

I was a chubby kid who spent most nights in front of the TV with ice cream and candy. My mom always told me to "Never make fun of the fat kids at school." Maybe that's why I felt a special affinity for this newcomer.

Or maybe it was because I knew his life was about to get even more miserable than it was before he took this job. Working in the advertising department at Macy's at the time was a pretty dismal way to make a living. Both Gregg and I knew we had to make some changes in our lives.

I watched Gregg transform into the super good-looking guy he is now, the person he actually always was, just a much healthier version that doesn't have to pay for an extra airplane seat or that mean kids or superficial coworkers snicker at or don't want to bother with anymore.

I, too, decided to remove the toxicity from my life, so I quit the awful world of corporate America, packed my bags and moved to Italy. That time period seems like 100 years ago. But, fortunately for me, Gregg is still a part of my life.

What Gregg did with his body and his life is astounding, and he continues to inspire me every day.

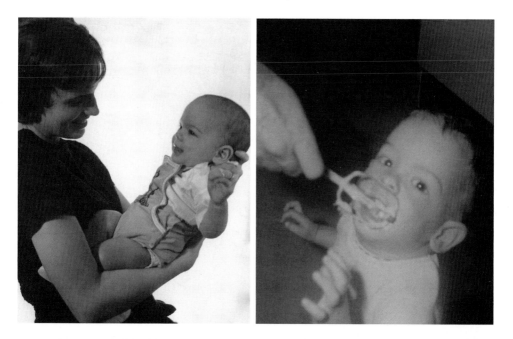

A NEW **STAR** iS BORN!

Presenting the "main attraction" at our house....

Star's Name *William Bragg*

Date of Debut *March 5th*

Weighed *8 lbs. 6 oz.*

Supporting Cast

Diana + Bill McBride

Top: Given my penchant for being a ham, I think the birth announcement my mother chose is quite appropriate. And making my debut at eight-pounds-and-six-ounces was something I didn't mind having in print, as opposed to documenting my excessive weight in later years.

Bottom left: I find this picture of my mom holding infant me fascinating. What was the woman who would go to her grave claiming I was adopted thinking when she looked into my eyes?

Bottom right: As far as I'm concerned, this shot of my dad letting me lick the batter off of a mixer attachment is proof that none of my eventual weight gain was my fault. (Yes, I'm kidding, but still!)

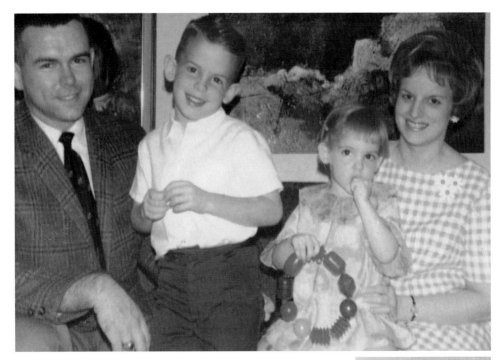

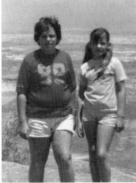

Top: Our family portrait. This was right about the time things started to unravel. You can read my sister Lori's take on our childhood beginning on page 19.

Right: Lori and I on a cross-country trip we took before moving to Singapore. I'm not sure which is more embarrassing about this photo— my growing belly or my short-shorts.

Bottom right: Despite being embarrassed by my excessive weight, if there were ever a photo opportunity to be had with high school kids I deemed "popular and attractive," I would always jump into the frame. I barely knew these people at the time this photo was taken.

Bottom left: Soda was always a staple of mine. I remember when I was very young I could barely drink a whole can by myself. But by the time I was a freshman in high school (seen here), I could polish off more than a six-pack all on my own.

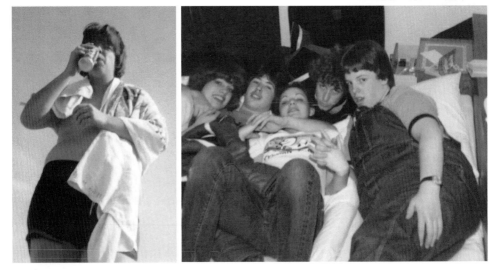

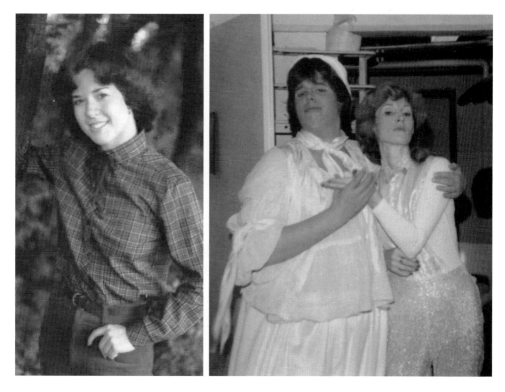

Top left: This is Amy, my girlfriend in high school (the one who had to suffer through my movie theater seat breaking debacle). You can read Amy's account of this incident beginning on page 44.

Top right: Here I am hamming it up backstage with one of the many friends I met while doing community theater in Wiesbaden, Germany. This is Vickie, the friend who, like everyone else, assumed that my mom couldn't possibly be lying about me being adopted and that I must have been the one with the problem since I "didn't want to admit it was true."

Bottom: These three pictures capture my mother's metamorphosis into "Dee-ana" perfectly. The first pic is my mom before getting married, the second is my mom while I was in high school (when she was married to my dad), and the third was taken while she was married to her second husband, Joe.

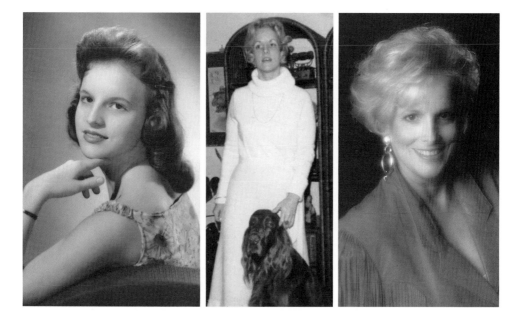

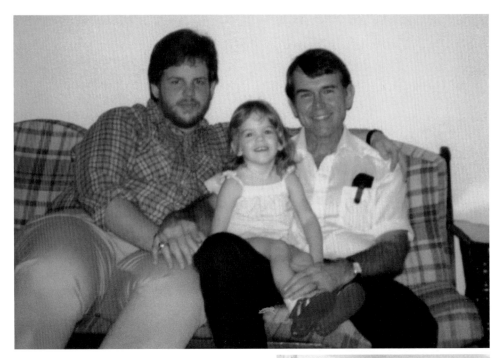

Top: Here I am with my dad and Nicole, his daughter and my half-sister.

Right: Here I am while attending Lynn University, having not only grown a beard (in an effort to emphasize my being a male despite my man boobs), but where I also created a kitchenette in my dorm room so that I could prepare and eat food in private 24/7.

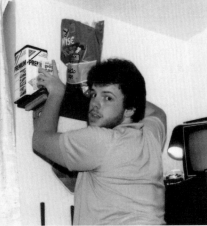

Bottom right: Here I am with my friend Erika while attending Florida State University. I'm wearing the oversized shirt that I "won" at the college bookstore after the manager displayed it as a joke, offering to give it away to whomever it fit. You can read what it was like for Erika to witness this exchange beginning on page 72.

Bottom left: One Halloween, I decided to make the most of my size. So I went to a costume party as The Love Boat (yes, I dressed up as the actual ship). Ever the good sport, my friend Elizabeth dressed up as regular Love Boat guest star, Charo.

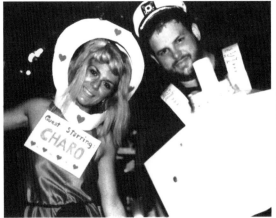

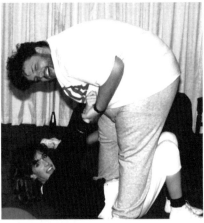

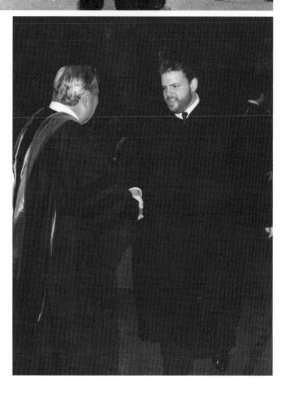

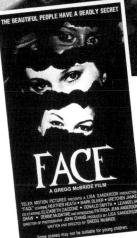

Top: That's me, far right, doing my best impression of Alfred Hitchcock on the set of one of the student films I directed while attending FSU. Here we were shooting a scene from a script I wrote called *Face*, about a beautiful co-ed who becomes the obsession of her fellow students.

Bottom right: Attending the graduation ceremony at FSU was one of the most difficult things I've ever done, mentally. I felt like the whole world was aghast at my size. No family or friends were there to see me get my diploma, but I still wanted to receive it publicly. Looking back, this was probably one of the bravest things I ever did.

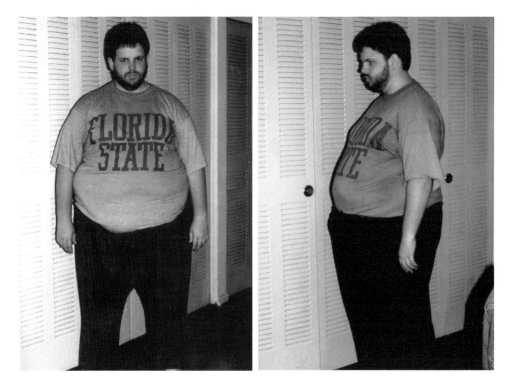

Top: Even though I had tried virtually hundreds of diets up until this time, I was still determined to take off the excess weight. So I had my friend Elizabeth take these "Before Pictures." I remember that while the pictures were being taken, the elastic waistband of the sweatpants was "eating" into my waist. As soon as these images were captured, I had to take them off and put on my bathrobe for relief.

Bottom: Here I am with my friend Kim at one of my student film premiers. What should have been an exciting night was marred by the fact that my clothes were so tight they were literally cutting off my circulation.

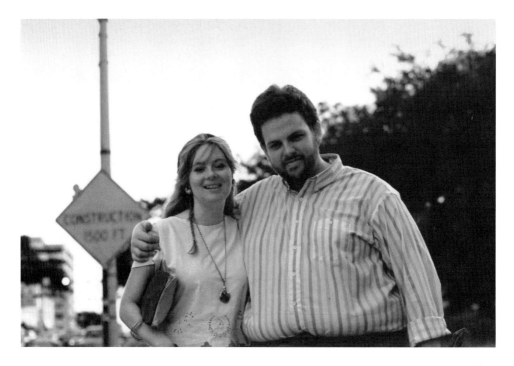

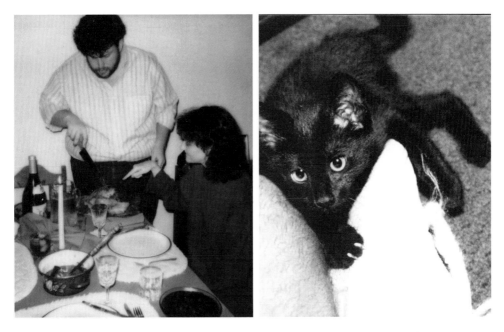

Top left: Despite being from a broken family, I was always desperate to create "family-like" scenarios. This meant cooking on one Thanksgiving for my boss (and friend) Donna and her niece. I wanted everything to be perfect. If only I could breathe in the pants I was wearing (I couldn't). You can read Donna's account of this beginning on page 103.

Top right: This is my cat Shadow, who literally loved me through thick and through thin. I credit her with the reason I'm alive today, since when planning to kill myself, I was so worried about her safety and who and when someone would find her that I decided not to go through with it.

Bottom: This shot was taken during one of my visits to see Kathi-Jo in New Orleans. During this time period I was convinced that Kathi-Jo didn't want to be seen with me in public because of my gargantuan size. Even so, I felt like if I could capture some visual memories with the "beautiful people," it somehow validated me as a person. You can read Kathi-Jo's account of this time in our lives beginning on page 69.

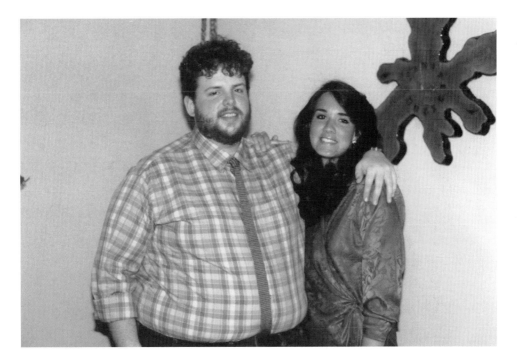

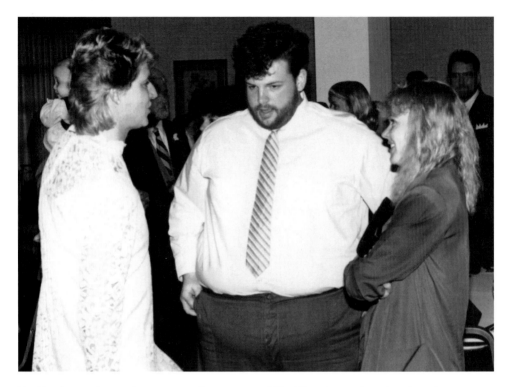

Top: Here I am busting out of my pants, standing near my good friend Kim who experienced people staring at us because of my size—trying to figure out why a thin girl was with a guy who was so heavy. You can read Kim's reaction to peoples' stares beginning on page 243.

Bottom right: Joining Weight Watchers in the Kansas City area turned out to be a major blessing in the form of one Petra—someone who is still a good friend to this day. Nothing bonds a friendship like cheating on your diets together. You can read Petra's account of our Weight Watchers adventures beginning on page 105.

Bottom left: Having relocated to the Kansas City area after college, I was ready to find a full-time job. Here I am in my "Big and Tall Store best"—ready for my interviews. Little did I know that getting a job while at this size was going to be incredibly difficult.

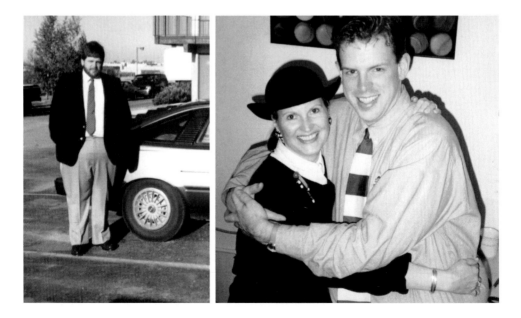

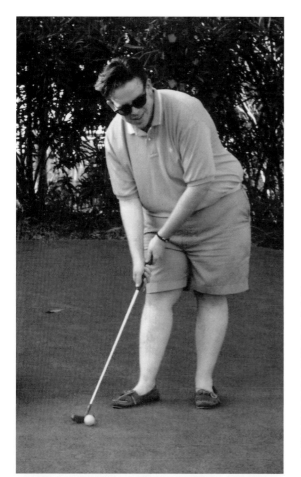

Left: There was nothing "miniature" about me during the time this shot was taken. Note the designer "average-sized people" shoes—the only apparel items I could purchase outside of a Big and Tall Store.

Bottom: Moving to the New York metropolitan area meant getting part-time work at The Cat's Pyjamas gift shop. Owners Gail (far right) and her partner Michael (who we're holding) never seemed to mind my excessive weight. My friend Elizabeth ended up getting a job at the store, too. And it was here that I met my longtime friend, Sally (far left). You can read Sally's account of our working together at this store beginning on page 123.

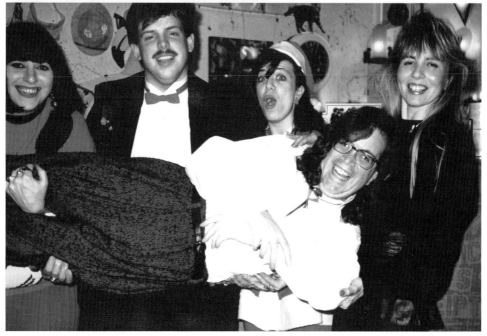

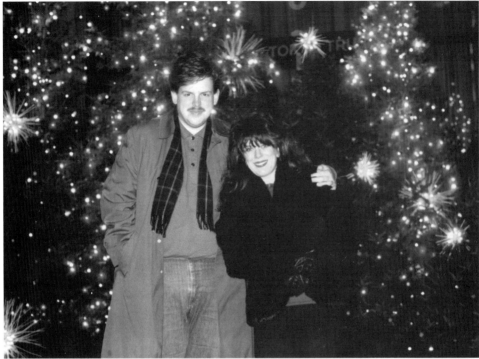

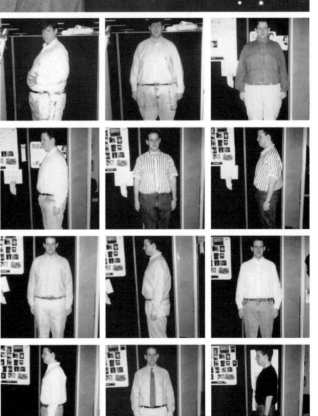

Top: Here I am with Elizabeth (who I'd known since FSU) in NYC at Christmas time. Because my weight kept me single and because she was the "other woman" in her relationship, we "dated" each other to fill in all of our alone time.

Bottom right: After starting work at Macy's and having a few mental breakthroughs, I finally started to really take off the excess weight once and for all. My progress was documented via Polaroid pictures week after week.

Bottom left: Here it is—my sixty-inch belt, which I've kept as a memento to this day. You can see where the belt was stretching out on the left. Even at sixty inches, I was having trouble getting it around my waist while at my heaviest weight.

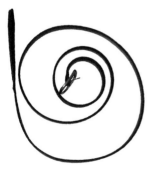

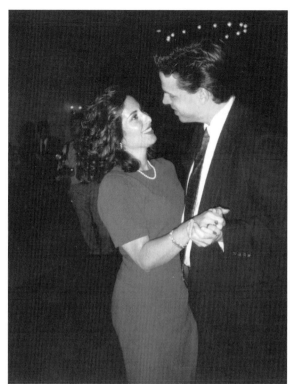

Left: Here I am with my fellow Macy's cohort Charlene. You can read Charlene's take on my journey from "before" to "after" and our time together working at Macy's beginning on page 143.

Bottom: My move to San Francisco was a result of securing a copywriting gig at an advertising agency in Marin County. Here I am with art director Rita, who always told it like it was. You can read Rita's account of me putting back on a lot of the weight that I'd lost beginning on page 157.

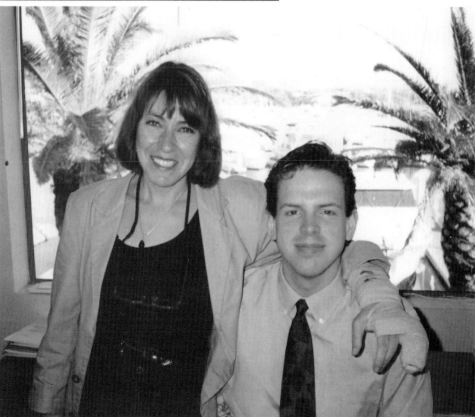

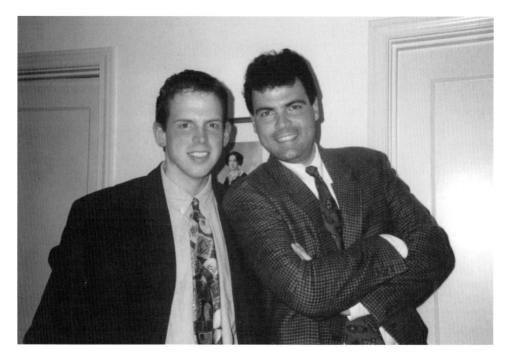

Top: While living in San Francisco I regained around 100 pounds of the 250 pounds of excess weight that I initially lost. It was mortifying to go back up the scale after having achieved so much success. Here I'm seen with my roommate, Nik. You can read Nikolai's account of my skin reduction surgery beginning on page 192.

Bottom: I finally managed to take most of the re-gained 100 pounds off. I was still insecure though—and that meant always wanting to pose with the "beautiful people." I'm seen here with two people from the SF advertising agency, art director Linda and account manager Cindy. You can read Linda's take on my obsession with the "beautiful people" beginning on page 174.

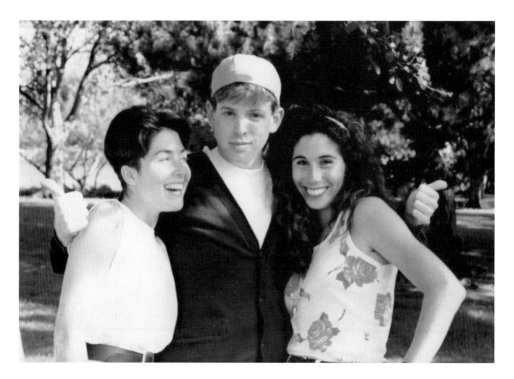

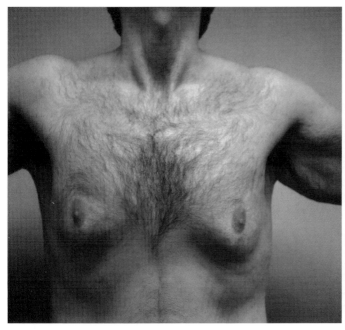

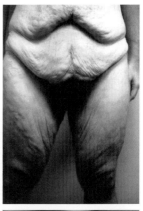

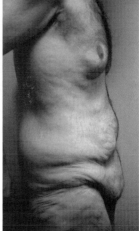

Top and right: My plastic surgeon took these "before surgery" pictures to document the amount of excess skin he was going to be taking off. At the time the pictures were taken, I swore I would never show them to anyone. The doctor ended up cutting away over a yard and a half of loose skin.

Bottom: Los Angeles. Here I am post skin-reduction surgery with professional model Ulli who worked for me while I was a freelance art director and eventually became a good friend. You can read Ulli's account of calling me on my "bullshit" beginning on page 213.

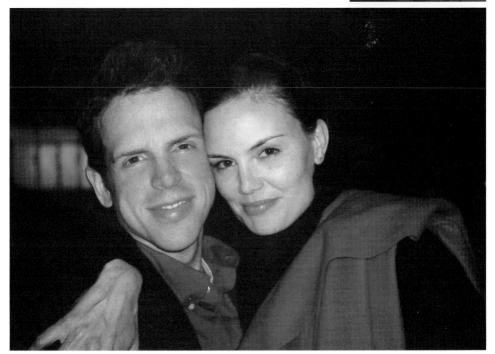

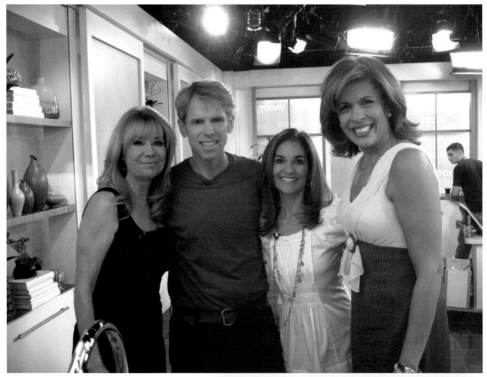

Top: Appearing on NBC's *Today* show and meeting Kathie Lee Gifford and Hoda Kotb was a blast. And I joked with nutrition expert Joy Bauer that meeting her was like meeting the rock star of dieting gurus. Joy is not only an amazing inspiration, but also has become a very good friend. Joy graciously wrote the Foreword to this book, which you can read beginning on page ix.

Right and facing page: Even now it's not that often that I take my shirt off in public. Despite weighing around 175 pounds, I'm still very self-conscious about my body and about feeling judged.

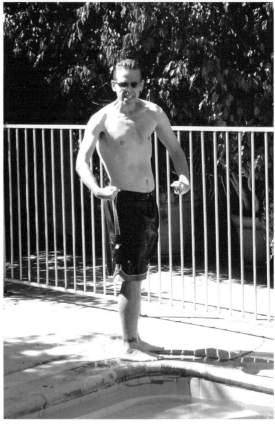

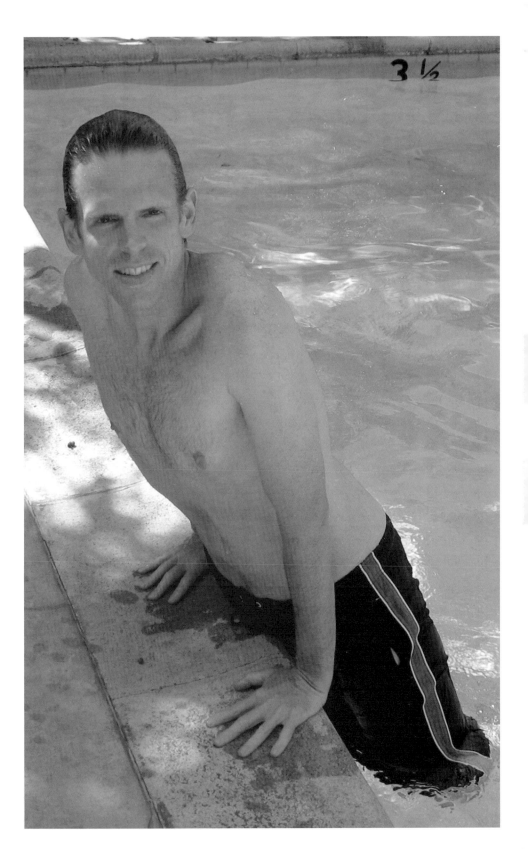

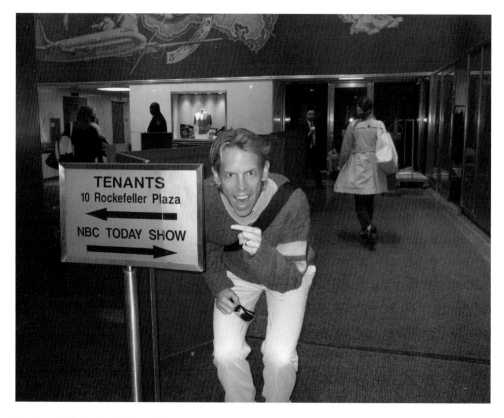

Top: I was thrilled to be asked to make another appearance on the *Today* show to help promote Joy Bauer's latest book release.

Bottom: Here I am today with my seven-pound bundle of unconditional love and my own little Zen master, Latte.

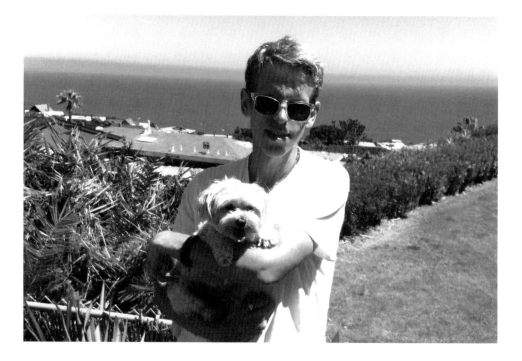

CHAPTER SEVEN

rise and fall

It was now approximately one year after I'd begun my latest diet. And to my, and everyone else's, surprise, I had taken off nearly 250 pounds almost to the day when I'd started it. When I share that fact today—that releasing the excess weight took no more than a year—people don't believe me and start asking which diet pill I took or which surgeon I saw for a gastric bypass. When I confirm that none of those methods were used, they start asking where I keep the magic wand.

I know it's a jaw-dropping fact that I took off so much weight in a seemingly short amount of time. You and I know that it was through careful eating, healthy amounts of exercise, drinking lots of water, and getting plenty of sleep. But no one wants to hear that. They want the magic wand explanation. Then they want to know where they can buy the magic wand.

You probably realize by now that my story doesn't end here. Otherwise this would be the epilogue and it's most definitely *not*.

Soon after reaching my goal weight of 185 pounds, I started hearing words I never imagined I would: "Gregg, do you think you're getting a little too skinny?" I was flattered. I was thrilled. I was a little out of touch. I couldn't believe I was getting that kind of attention.

When I weighed in excess of 400 or even 450 pounds no one wanted to talk about my weight issues. But now that I was borderline "too skinny," it was *all* anyone wanted to talk about. And I have to admit I loved being in the spotlight for what I thought were all the right reasons.

So much so that I didn't alter my diet at all once I reached my final goal weight. In fact, I started eating a little less than I had been on a daily basis. It was all very subconscious. Now that I was at what society considered a "normal weight," I was suddenly much busier, socially speaking. I was only too happy to make plans after work, join friends for a drink, or even hit a club to go dancing. This kind of life was all very new to me. And I wanted to go anywhere I could to show off my new "average-sized" clothes.

This new schedule meant very little time at home. I was still commuting from New Jersey to NYC for work, and was only getting a few hours of sleep a night. I blamed my poor eating habits on the shorter amounts of time I had for meal preparation.

Shadow pooping in my bed should have been a sign that I wasn't going about things in the healthiest of ways. According to friends who knew more about feline behavior than I did, my cat was sending me a message that I wasn't home enough. Shadow was used to me being a virtual recluse outside of working hours, but now I was never home. Of course I made sure she had food, water, and a clean litter box. But my full-time attention had been reduced to less than part-time. It must have been a tough thing for her to adjust to.

But even Shadow's stinky message didn't get through to me. Not in regard to my ridiculous schedule or "need" to be liked or my current eating habits.

A Typical Day of Gregg's Post-Weight-Loss Eating

BREAKFAST

1 cup All-Natural Cereal (like Kashi)

½ cup of 2% Reduced Fat Milk

½ of a medium Banana, sliced into chunks and mixed with the cereal

LUNCH

Lunch Salad

6 oz. of Broiled Chicken, chopped into chunks

2 cups Fresh Cherry Tomatoes, sliced in half

Balsamic Vinegar and Fresh Ground Pepper

EVENING SNACK

A cocktail or two (usually consumed right after work)

DINNER

1 piece of Fruit (usually eaten just before bed)

Before too long people were telling me my face was looking gaunt. The ever-subtle Charlene took to calling me "Skeletor." In my twisted brain I took this all as a weird compliment, all to somehow let me know that I was on the right track.

I wasn't trying to hurt myself or to get "extra skinny." But that's what was happening. I realized that my face was caving in on itself, but I was focused on my waistline, which continued to stall out at a thirty-eight inch waist. I wanted it to be smaller. I had seen an episode of *Seinfeld,* in which the character played by Jerry Seinfeld was caught changing the waist size on his jeans from a thirty-two to a thirty-one. I decided that thirty-one inches was the waist size I needed to have, not realizing that besides having a different metabolism than Jerry Seinfeld, I had mounds and mounds of loose skin to contend with.

Even though I was now under my goal weight, I still wasn't comfortable with my body. I had stretch marks all over my chest, stomach, back, upper arms, and upper thighs. I also had super baggy, saggy skin. I exercised at least three times a week and ate very nutritionally while losing the excess weight, but I still had enough skin to cover a 450 pound body. Turns out that no matter how much exercise you do, most of the excess skin will not retract.

This is something that isn't often spoken or written about in weight loss circles. I was wearing "clothes sizes that thin people wear," but I had to fold layers of skin into my pant legs and shirtsleeves.

On top of that, I had to be very careful about the kind of shirt material I wore. If the material was too thin or translucent, anyone would be able to see my saggy man boobs. While there was no more fat making them stick out like a pair of women's breasts, the saggy sacks that used to hold my man boobs were still there. I did everything I could to hide them from the world.

In hindsight, I may have reduced my calorie intake even after reaching my goal weight in order to combat the loose skin. Also in hindsight, my unhealthy eating habits I developed after taking the excess weight off only made the loose skin worse. I wasn't getting the nutrients I needed and as a result my skin looked pasty and unhealthy. My energy level was at an all-time low. Even my hair started to thin out. After a year-long attempt to get and be healthy, I'd accomplished anything but that.

With that new lack of energy came a really crappy work ethic. I was phoning in my copywriting assignments at Macy's, and Joan, my boss, was hip to my dysfunction. Joan now saw me as a party boy rather than a hard worker.

I was falling from grace. *Fast.*

Others in the advertising department weren't as quick to see this decline, but still, I knew the time was nigh to get out of Dodge, i.e., Macy's.

Looking back, I realize I should have risen to the occasion and reminded Joan of what kind of dynamic ad writer I could be. But I was like a kid in a candy store, too enamored with my new "social life of a thin person." I wasn't willing to trade anything for that, not my career or, as it turns out, my self-respect.

When I set out to find a new job I never imagined I would end up in San Francisco. I had never even visited before. But a friend at Macy's told me about a small advertising agency that was looking for a temporary copywriter, offering a three-month contract with the possibility of going full-time, so I decided to throw my hat into the ring.

This was the first time I was interviewing in a suit purchased from an "average sizes" clothing store. Kate, the copy director at the agency who interviewed me, was impressed with my copywriting work as well as my sense of humor.

There I was at a job interview not worrying about being dismissed as soon as the interviewer saw my size. Even though I was being interviewed by a woman, and knowing women had often been more empathetic toward me when I was heavy than men, it was still surreal. Not only did Kate make eye contact with me, I also didn't have to hold in my stomach. Those were things I'd never experienced during the job interviewing process before. I also didn't need to control my labored breathing. And thanks to the suit jacket covering things up, I didn't worry about my loose skin creating weird patterns under my clothing. I was hired for the three-month period, but Kate secretly knew she would be leaving the company in the fall to have a baby. I didn't know of her plans at the time, but I was thrilled when I was offered a full-time position with the firm at the end of my temporary tenure.

SAN FRANCISCO HERE I COME

As I prepared to leave New York City, I decided I would leave Shadow behind as well. My girlfriend from high school, Amy (who now lived in the metro Washington, DC area), agreed to adopt Shadow and take care of her. Amy is a big animal advocate, so I knew Shadow would be in good hands.

I thought I was doing the right thing by giving Shadow to Amy. I hoped that my busy social life would continue and knew I'd be living with a friend temporarily when first arriving to the Bay Area. But honestly, I still carry a lot of remorse over that decision to this day. Shadow had been a dedicated ally during my heavy years when it seemed few in the human world wanted anything to do with me. So the minute I became what I thought was accepted by the "real world," I sent Shadow to a new home. I'm sure she was confused. Clearly I was as well.

Life in San Francisco was very different from life on the East Coast. Before leaving for the Bay Area, I had moved into New York City for a few months. Without a car, the city can really make one feel boxed in, especially during winter. So arriving in San Francisco during the month of May was a breath of fresh air, literally.

The most exciting part of starting the new job was the beginning of what I considered my brand new life. No one at this agency knew that I used to tip the scales at over 450 pounds. I loved that I had a secret of sorts and felt as if I were playing a role on some prime time soap opera of "thin, cool Gregg." No longer did I need to be "foxy for a fat kid."

I can see now that I hadn't yet come together as a whole person. Just as society seemed to view me only in terms of "before-and-after," so was I seeing myself. I continued to live and be somewhat out of touch, socially—treating people more like objects rather than human beings.

My social awkwardness was a true Achilles' heel when dealing with friends just as it was when interacting with potential paramours.

As clumsy as I was out on the dance floor at clubs, I was even clumsier when dating. About five minutes into every first date, no matter who it was with, I would decide "This is the one" and immediately fall in love. I wouldn't hold back communicating my fervent adoration either, which usually meant there were very few second dates.

What's wrong with these people? I thought to myself. *Don't they realize I'm thin now and they should be falling in love with me?*

Oh. So. Very. Confused.

Meanwhile, at the new advertising agency, I longed to be part of the "in" crowd. I still saw all social situations as the high school cafeteria of life.

Because our offices were located in Sausalito the agency had a giant sailboat at the nearby dock, which the two owners would use to take visiting clients out on. A select few from the creative staff would be invited to go along sailing, out into the bay, underneath the Golden Gate Bridge and back to the pier outside of our offices.

Linda Souders was one such member of the creative staff. With her pixie haircut, model-like looks, and incredible artistic talent, she seemed to be the belle of the ball. Turns out Linda was very much in touch with her holistic side as well. She was a big fan of self-awareness and didn't seem to be buying into my overactive "let's be best friends instantly" banter for one second.

Linda's office was upstairs along with those of the other creative elites', on the main floor of the agency. I was relegated to the bottom floor offices, a windowless area divided into small cubicles where freelancers also happened to work.

One such freelancer was brassy, sassy, and oh-so-real Rita Wood. Rita was an art director originally from the East Coast who never minced words. If she thought it, she said it. I used to wince and hold my breath when I heard her being direct with people at the agency, even the owners. I marveled at her audacity to tell it like it is and be completely honest.

Honesty? Is she nuts? There's no place for honesty in advertising.

Rita also saw through my attempts at sitting at the cool kids' table, all the way to my layers of desperation and hidden loose skin. She saw a real person waiting to be discovered.

Rita constantly called me out on my lame efforts to fit in. She wouldn't let one awkward attempt to be cool slip by, unless it was authentic. And it never really was. I realize now that I was still in high school mode, that is, always clowning around, always telling jokes, and always working too hard to be accepted in order to feel loved.

Had this been a *Star Wars* movie, this is the scene in which Yoda might have appeared to tell me that "For true acceptance, on the inside must you look." But Yoda wasn't around, just Linda, and the other beautiful art directors who seemed to be shunning me.

It was just around this time that I was assigned to write copy for the Ethel M Chocolates account, a chocolatier out of Nevada that specialized in gourmet chocolate treats in a variety of "creamy, crunchy, and chewy assortments."

Twice a year, boxes and boxes and boxes of every kind of chocolate one can imagine were shipped to our agency where, on the ground level (where my cubicle and the agency's photo studio happened to be), they would be photographed for catalogs and other forms of print advertising. This meant that for about thirty days, two times a year, the agency hallways were overflowing with decadent chocolate.

Once the chocolates were photographed or had been passed over by photography due to slight visual imperfections, they ended up in the break room, where anyone at the agency could enjoy a piece or two—and do so while complaining they were breaking their diet no matter how much they did or didn't weigh.

But not me. I was specially trained in the high stakes world of snacking. I knew how to get a bounty of chocolate out of the break room without being noticed, therefore not having to say anything about dieting, since those people didn't even know the "fat me" ever existed.

I would walk into the break room with a large plastic bag and empty a tray or two of chocolate into it, resulting in me ending up with one to two pounds of chocolate. I would then take said bag back down to my cubicle, position it behind my computer monitor, and proceed to nibble from it throughout the day.

If by chance someone popped their head into my area and saw me chewing a piece of chocolate, I would tell them I was tasting it so that I would know how to write about it (*uh-huh*). But as soon as they disappeared, I would scoop another piece (or four) into my mouth.

Little did I know I had fallen back into an old coping mechanism. If I couldn't get love from Linda or the other popular creative folks on staff, then I was going to get love from Ethel M's Almond Butter Crisps, Almond Crunch Dark Chocolates, Almond Clusters, Pecan Toffee Crisps, and well, the list goes on.

A Typical Day of Gregg's Eating in San Francisco

BREAKFAST

1 Fast Food "Egg" (or resembling such) Sandwich

1 large 7–11 Coffee (with heavy, flavored Cream)

LUNCH

2 slices of Pizza

Side Salad with bottled Italian Dressing

2–3 Diet Cokes

AFTERNOON SNACK

20 to 40 pieces of Chocolate

(Crème, Nut, Caramel, Truffle, and Solid Varieties)

DINNER

Broiled Chicken (without skin)

Steamed Vegetables

Water

I'm not aware of exactly how it happened. Surely I had to have changed pant sizes a couple of times throughout the process. But one day I woke up, realizing I'd put on quite a bit of weight.

This was further emphasized when Rita came into the office after she'd been away for several weeks, took one look at me and plainly announced, "You got fat."

I was floored by her rudeness or rather, her honesty.

Searching for a clever response, I had none. I could feel my face turning eight shades of red knowing good and well she was right—I had gained weight (something I hadn't even considered admitting to myself until that moment). I quickly scurried past Rita, into the photo studio, where I knew there happened to be a scale.

When I stepped onto the scale, my eyes must have popped out of my head cartoon-style, like those belonging to an animated mouse seeing a menacing cat.

I weighed around 285 pounds.

Since the last time I had really checked in with my weight (*really really* checked in), I had gained 100 pounds.

Suddenly it all made sense. No wonder my pants were so tight (the two pair of pants I could fit into). No wonder I was popping buttons on my dress shirts, hidden by ties I wore to mask how they were battling to keep my shirt fastened over my growing belly. No wonder I was often sweaty and out-of-breath. I had gained 100 pounds.

Gained. Yeah, right.

I couldn't believe it. I had become another conformer to the diet industry statistic, which dictates that most people who lose large amounts weight gain the same amount, if not more of it, back.

I had to admit defeat as I became sick of mending clothes that were ripping from being stretched onto my body for hours at a time and creating holes in the inside thighs of my pant legs from my thighs constantly rubbing together, I had to research the nearest Big and Tall clothing store and make the drive there. I had grown to a fifty-two-inch waist.

One of the worst things about wearing a size fifty-two-inch waist again was realizing that the last time I had worn that size, I had been jubilant. I had been wearing a sixty-inch waist at my all-time high. So getting down to a fifty-two-inch waist was cause for celebration. But there I was back at the same fifty-two inches again. Clearly, that was not celebration-worthy.

People at the agency stared at me. They had no idea I had weighed over 450 pounds when I graduated from college. They only knew me as the semi-svelte copywriter they had hired less than a year before. I thought I could see both shock and pity in their eyes.

Yet as much as I was mortified, I was also somehow comfortable again. Yes. Comfortable.

Because "fat Gregg" was the Gregg I'd grown up with.

The Gregg I knew.

The Gregg who had an excuse to hide from the world and not attempt to spread his wings.

The Gregg who could complain about his abusive parents who never called, wrote, or took an interest in his life.

The Gregg who could blame his nonexistent love life on being too heavy to take his clothes off.

The Gregg whose only real friend was a cat. A cat he had left behind.

But not even Shadow was there for me now. In fact, news had come from Amy that Shadow had gone through some terrible medical issues and that Amy had to ultimately make the very tough decision to allow Shadow to pass away.

Instead of feeling sorry for Shadow or for Amy, who was heartbroken, not to mention broke due to the high vet bills, I felt sorry for myself. "How could this happen to *me*?" I lamented. With a fifty-two-inch going on a fifty-four-inch waist, I may not have been the fattest person in the world, but I certainly might have been the most selfish.

After a particularly gluttonous binge, during which I stuffed so much food down my throat I was laying on the floor in agony, I woke up in the middle of the night, covered in sweat. I tried to drink a little water to fight the heartburn, but only ended up throwing up some of the food that was still processing in my over-filled stomach.

Stumbling to the bathroom, I stood over the sink, splashing water onto my face, trying to cool myself down. I felt feverish and sick.

It was dark, but I caught a good glimpse of myself in the mirror. There he was.

Fat Gregg.

Puffy cheeks.

Sweaty forehead.

Bewildered gaze.

Panting and out-of-breath.

Heart beating too fast.

T-shirt and underwear cutting into fleshy stomach and thighs.

And yet . . . I saw something more.

Looking into my eyes, I suddenly got in touch with the fact that I'd handled Shadow's death and Amy's grief over the incident in a very self-absorbed way. I also realized that I'd been putting on airs at work, trying to get certain people to like me no matter what I had to do to accomplish it, just to further my own social standing.

After a long, labored breath, I spoke out loud to my reflection in the mirror.

"Congratulations," I said with a hint of irony. "You've become your mother."

ANOTHER PERSPECTIVE ON GREGG AT THIS TIME

By Rita Wood, Gregg's Coworker at the SF Agency

When Gregg first gave me these pages to read, it brought me to tears. I had no clue he was struggling so much with his demons during that time. As I read the words I felt increasingly awful, wondering if I could have helped or done something more—*anything*—to make his life a little easier. But I didn't realize what was going on at the time. His inner struggle was invisible. Gregg hid it well.

The incidents of which he speaks happened many years ago. To be honest, I have no memory of telling him he was fat. I certainly might have been kidding around, trying to keep it light in our dysfunctional workplace.

I liked Gregg from the minute we met. He was a fun work friend who didn't think he was writing some great American novel when copy for an ad needed to be edited, like some more pretentious copywriters did. He was a professional, and I respected that. His sense of humor was appreciated. Did I think he was fat? At the time I might have called him chubby, maybe a little fat, not huge, not abnormal. Of course, I didn't know he was once much fatter or thinner.

What Gregg doesn't mention is the type of work environment he found at that "direct marketing advertising agency" in Sausalito, California. If there were such a thing as a sweatshop for the college educated, this would be it. Young writers, artists, and account executives were hunched over their computers, churning out page after page of catalogs under impossible deadlines. Believe me, after my (then) twenty-year career in advertising, I knew this agency was exceptional in dishing out the stress. Twelve-hour days were routine. And yes, there were lots of food products for the clients' photo shoots. I remember management bringing in greasy pizza to the break room, midday, because no one ever had time to go to lunch.

Gregg and I were originally hired as extra sets of hands for the drowning-in-work, stressed-out white collar slaves. These were the folks Gregg refers to as the upstairs "in" people. I had a different view of the upstairs, downstairs thing.

Downstairs was a quiet place where Gregg and I were blessedly separated from the upstairs craziness, quietly tucked between the bookkeeper's office and a photo studio where we could toil in peace. Outdated computers and windowless rooms were small prices to pay to be at a safe distance from the beautiful people upstairs who handled their anxiety by doing lots of "stress-reducing substances" and screwing around behind their spouses' backs.

When we needed a break from the constant grind, we would wander into the photo studio where the tempting food products were awaiting their close-ups. The combination of proximity, stress, and no lunch break was the perfect storm for bad eating habits, even for us "thin" people. Everyone ate that damned chocolate, myself included. In fact, I had one of the worst acne breakouts of my life because of it. Everyone gained a few pounds. But for Gregg it must have been especially lethal.

CHAPTER EIGHT

trusting my inner dieter

Along with carrying around the extra 100 pounds I regained, I was also playing mind games with myself again. They consisted of "little tricks" I would use to try and stay on my diet and lose weight. The key word here was "tricks." And *tricks* tend to be just that: "A cunning or skillful act or scheme intended to deceive or outwit someone." Only my tricks were hardly cunning.

As many times as I attempted to restart the diet with which I'd lost the 250 pounds, I would counteract those efforts by sneaking back in what I wanted to eat. For example, I set a rule that I would "never eat any fattening foods or go off my diet while at home." Well, cut to me sitting in my parked car, eating bags full of fast food before going into my apartment building. I'd sit in the car, embarrassed whenever someone would drive or walk by. If I was in the middle of chewing, I would stop and hide whatever food I was eating until I was alone again.

Gregg's Typical Post-Diet Binge

1 Fast Food Hamburger

1 Fast Food Chicken Sandwich

1 medium order of Chicken Bites/Nuggets

1 order of Curly Fries

1 order of Onion Rings

2 large Sprites

1 Fruit Pie

1 large Chocolate Milkshake

I was once again consuming so much food it was deadening my senses. Coming home after eating enough for two to three people, I would stumble into the bathroom, splash water onto my sweating forehead, and then take off my clothes so I could wash them before the next business day. I had only one pair of pants that fit and only a couple of shirts I could button up. The shirts looked like they were ripping apart a la *The Incredible Hulk*, so I had to cover the centers of the shirts with a wide business dress tie.

After deciding that my old diet wasn't "working," I turned to the many wacky or faddy diets available. As before, I would only make it about six to twelve hours on any given diet, only to give up, deciding to try again the next day (or, if it was Wednesday or Thursday, the Monday of the following week) and then to succumb to whatever food I was craving.

I was actively partaking in what those of us with a dieter's mentality call the "last supper syndrome." This phenomenon happens when a dieter thinks he or she can never have a certain type of food again. So, in order to counteract that, we eat as much of said food as we can as a "last supper" before beginning a diet or new way of life.

Sick. Silly. Sad. Mind games. Plain and simple.

This "last supper" behavior results in a vicious on-off cycle that is one of the most damning aspects of the dieter's mentality. When we're "on" a diet, we are too good, to the extremes of feeling deprived. And when we're "off" our diets, we take it to the extremes as well. The extremes of overeating. Coworkers at the advertising agency were looking at me out of the corners of their eyes. They were in awe of the fact that I put on 100 pounds as quickly as I did. If I caught the stares, I would tell them that I used to weigh more than this current weight and that I was just going through a period of adjustment. I would then usually reveal a baggie with carrot sticks in it as if to prove that I had the situation handled.

Meanwhile, I'd be scouring the company break room for any remnants of Ethel M candy or any other food product we might have had on hand as a result of our doing an advertising campaign. This would include eating our client's Knott's Berry Farms preserves and jams directly out of the jars as if they were pudding cups. I was now afraid to even sneak eat those foods in the confines of my cubicle, so I once again took my secret binge edibles into the bathroom.

There I was, just as I had been in college, sitting in a toilet stall, munching down on whatever fattening food products I could find. Anytime someone came into the bathroom I would stop chewing and hold my breath—waiting for them to take care of "business," wash their hands, and depart so that my bathroom binge could continue.

No matter how much eating I did, I could not shake the image I had come face to face with weeks before, feeling like I was staring back at my mother when I looked into a mirror.

I had very little contact with my mother or father at that time. It was as if moving to the West Coast had given me an excuse not to be in touch with them. I told myself that was all very healthy, mentally. Yet there I was, eating to the point of pain and excess (once again), while also attempting to live some kind of façade in order to get Linda and the other "pretty people" at the agency to like and accept me.

The thought of having morphed into my mother, who had also done anything at all costs to attain her idea of popularity, was an unsettling one. I knew that was *not* the direction I wanted to continue in. I saw the kind of existence my mom had lived during the past two decades—an empty one full of lies and deceit, and one that always resulted in her losing friends once they found out they'd been deceived.

Gaining that clarity was earth-shattering to me, and not in a bad way.

For the first time, I didn't see my mom as the all-out enemy. While I never talked about my mom much to other people (being too embarrassed about the childhood I had lived through), I always had considered her the villain and the reason why I had to walk around with an inches-thick layer of blubber in order to protect myself from society's ills. Pretty convenient, right?

As I finally clarified the excuse that I'd kept just below the surface but that I had clearly been operating on as a result of thinking it, I realized that it was just *that*—an *excuse*. With these new and somewhat confusing thoughts filling my head, I decided to do something I hadn't done in a while—seek out some therapy. My health insurance at the time didn't cover much counseling, only a certain number of pre-approved visits a year. And very few visits at that. What's more, I had to call my provider and explain why I needed therapy. For some reason, that was a very embarrassing thing to do.

The insurance rep couldn't quite wrap her head around what I was trying to explain about what I was going through; however, she did caution me that eating disorders were not covered by my insurance plan. I suppose she pointed this out so that I would know to not emphasize my weight issues when filling out insurance forms so that I would, therefore, be approved to see a therapist.

DEAR MOM

I went to my first meeting with my appointed therapist, and I hated him.

Having had mostly women as friends and confidants throughout my life, I was put off by the fact that he was male. I also didn't like that he never laughed at my jokes and that he always had a stoic expression on his face whenever I explained some of the circumstances of my upbringing. Where was this guy's compassion? Didn't he know I was a *victim* and unable to help myself? That none of this was my fault? That all of this was my mother's fault?

After the first visit, I decided I wasn't going to go back to him. I also decided that I wasn't going to read the book he assigned me, *How to Stubbornly Refuse to Make Yourself Miserable about Anything—Yes, Anything!* by Albert Ellis, PhD, and that I wasn't going to do my homework assignment of writing my mom a letter that explained how I felt about our shared past.

Instead, I drove to the nearest fast food place, went through the drive through, ordered enough for four people, then parked, sat in my car, and ate until my stomach hurt. Then, almost as if on auto pilot, I shifted the car into drive, drove to a bookstore, and bought the book I was never going to read.

As I grudgingly read the book, only to prove to myself how inappropriate it was for me to read it, I loathed every word. I didn't like its style of writing and I certainly didn't appreciate the author's "in your face" message that the emotional baggage I was carrying around was not anyone's fault in particular.

How could it not be my mother's fault? She's the one who did it to me and my sister!

Yes, I was arguing with the book but reading it nonetheless.

Along with reading (and hating) the book, I also decided to complete the homework assignment that I was never going to do. I wrote the letter to my mother that the therapist had asked me to write.

At my next appointment (the one I was never going to keep), I was asked to read the letter to my mother out loud. And so I did.

Dear Mom,

I am not exactly sure why I'm writing this letter. I'm not even sure I'm ever going to send it. But I wanted you to know some of the things I am feeling. So at the very least, I'll commit them to paper before deciding whether or not to actually mail this to you.

It may surprise you to know that even though I'd lost most of my excess weight while on the East Coast, I have now put over half of the weight back on. Obviously, I'm aware that this happened as a result of my overeating—and not because I have some mysterious disease that makes me fat (the disease you told your husband that I have). I'm fat because I eat. And I eat for protection.

In case you're wondering what I need protection from, well, that would be YOU.

It was so easy when Lori and I were younger to blame Dad for our miserable childhoods. Dad was never around, was always drinking, was more interested in dating flight attendants than being at our school functions, and was always anxious to handle any family upheaval with his belt, rather than through listening or talking.

But I now realize that although Dad shares in the responsibility as to what went on in our lives, much of the responsibility falls onto your shoulders. And if you think I'm pointing a finger here, you're right.

I'm not sure if you're still reading this. I know you have a habit of being very defensive and looking away from anything that doesn't fit into your little plan of how life should be or how the world should see you.

As your "adopted son" (and I know I'm not really adopted), I have to say that it really hurt, while growing up, to have my friends try to convince me that it was "okay" to be adopted and that I didn't have to lie to cover it up. That's how good your lies were, Mom. People believed you instead of your kids.

I remember one time when you, Joe, and I were driving somewhere together. We'd somehow gotten onto a conversation about babies. In fact, I think Joe was talking about his son as a baby. When Joe got out of the car for a minute, I remember asking you, "Mom, what were my first words?"

You snapped, replying "How should I know?" in a tone that was so dismissive I didn't dare pursue it (or any other conversation at the time) further. Even when we were alone you could not acknowledge me as your natural born son.

Thinking back to that situation, I am starting to realize that perhaps you believe your own lies more than anyone you tell the lies to. Why is that, Mom?

Do you really believe I am adopted?

Do you really believe that Lori is a drug addict?

Do you really see us as such threats that to admit you gave birth to us would be too much to bear?

Up until now I've not only played along with your lies, but I've also covered them up. With your employers. With your boyfriends. With your current husband. I've provided the perfect alibi for you. I've been the perfect partner in crime. And I'm realizing that now that I'm an adult, that saddles me with an equal share of the responsibility.

So today I'm going to take that responsibility one step further and ensure that the crimes (against me) will stop. I am no longer willing to play along. I am no longer willing to pretend. I will never again pick up the phone for you and pretend to be a female maid in order to keep your love life flowing smoothly.

I am your son. Not your adopted son. Your son. And I'm willing to talk more about this if you are, either over the phone or by letter. Your choice.

Love (yes, love),

Gregg

I looked up from my letter, prepared to see my normally nonplussed therapist bowled over in grief and empathy. Or, at the very least, bursting into applause given not only what I'd composed in my very poignant letter, but also for my award-worthy delivery. Instead, I was met with the same stoic face and a simple question.

"Do you want to mail the letter?"

Do I want to mail it? Yes, I want to mail it. I took the time to write it, didn't I?

The therapist then explained that writing the letter was more of an exercise for me, one in which I would hopefully be able to better clarify and articulate my own feelings. And I had to admit it had done just that.

But, of course, I still wanted to mail the letter. I was sure that my heartfelt prose would melt my mother's frozen heart and help her see the error of her horrific ways.

In other words, I wanted to be *right*.

My insurance only approved eight appointments with the therapist, so I was relieved when my mother wrote back as quickly as she did. When I received her reply I was anxious to share it with my therapist. At last, I had proof of my mother's conceit.

In her letter, she not only denied many of the things I accused her of (by not even addressing or acknowledging them), but also accused me of being the pathological liar and assuring me that she "warned" Joe that any contact I made personally with him should be ignored because of my psychosis.

My mother ended her letter by telling me how sorry she felt for me, and added that she hoped Lori and I would both eventually get the help we need.

My therapist was as unfazed by my mother's reply as he was by anything else I'd presented. He acknowledged that I *could* write her back, but mentioned that he didn't necessarily advise it, suggesting instead that I just *accept* who my mother is.

I was confounded by his suggestion. I felt that if I accepted who my mom was (and her resulting behavior) that I would not only be compliant with it, but virtually encouraging it.

The therapist helped me understand that I was compliant with it when assuming a female voice and playing social secretary for my mother; or when writing notes supposedly from my mother to teachers at school on Lori's behalf; or when making sure my sister and I were both dressed, fed, and got to school on time. He then pointed out that those acts were not only me being compliant, but me also being a survivalist. I did what I had to do to survive.

"And," he concluded, "perhaps that survival involved eating as well."

Had I not been sitting down I might have collapsed onto the floor. His words resonated inside me like a big church bell clanging at its loudest. I felt another rush of clarity that was almost freeing.

Nothing the therapist said, nothing I wrote, and nothing my mother wrote undid anything that had transpired before that moment. It had all happened. And no matter how unjust I thought it was, or how much I regretted some of my actions in the past (covering for my mom, overeating to compensate, trying desperately to get love from anyone I deemed to be one of the "beautiful people"), nothing was going to undo any of what had already taken place.

And that was okay *if* I was willing to let it be okay.

The first test of this kind of acceptance lay in the question of whether I wanted to write my mother back and counter everything she'd claimed in her letter to me. I definitely *wanted* to do that. But I also realized that it likely wouldn't do any good. And really, who cares if it did change her mind or not? I know what happened. So did Lori. And so did friends like Amy and others who could all wear T-shirts that proclaimed them "Diana survivors."

This was real. I was real. And, ultimately, that was then. And this was now. Forgive me if I fall into "bumper sticker-speak," but at that moment in my life I realized that, for me, that's really what it came down to. All of the current eating, current self-imposed loneliness, current fear, current shame, and current self-loathing was a result of what I was doing. Not what my mother was doing. Or even what she had done.

Still confused, and feeling a thousand emotions at once, I looked to the stoic therapist excitedly. I was ready for whatever was next in our therapy sessions. But that was when he closed his notebook and announced, "You don't need to see me anymore. You're *there*."

I wasn't buying it. I told him not only did I have two more sessions that were already pre-approved by my insurance, I was also anxious to get deeper into this.

"Why?" he asked. "Everything you need to know, you know."

I have to admit that it was some of the best (and toughest) therapy I'd ever received.

Up until that time, most of the "therapy" I'd had was the inadvertent kind through weight loss groups and other organizations that simply patted you on the back when you admitted that you cheated on your diet. A lot of "That's okay. You have an excuse."

Now? All my excuses seemed to have fallen away.

I'm not knocking whatever kind of therapy may work for someone else. But for me, this quick, tough love, rip-off-the-bandage-fast approach was really powerful.

For years I'd been listing all the reasons I had for overeating, hiding, hating myself, and doing things I thought would make other people like me.

At that moment, while sitting in the therapist's office, I was simply Gregg. The guy whose mom tells people he's adopted. And guess what? I'm not adopted. But who cares?

That was then. This is now.

Suddenly confronted by the "now," I knew I had 100-plus reasons (100 excess pounds) to eat healthier. But I also knew I needed to shift my approach to dieting just as I was learning to shift my approach regarding how I thought about my mom and my upbringing.

I called my sister, Lori, and tried to share the findings I'd made with the therapist's help with her. I probably came on a little too strong (think overly caffeinated cheerleader).

Lori wasn't too welcoming of my message to let the past, and Mom's abuse, go. Lori seemed to be carrying around a lot of her own hurt, a lot of pain, and a lot of scars. And she wasn't willing to give them up. So much so, that Lori, herself, was now morbidly obese. She had always been the thin sibling when we were younger. But I'm guessing the years of pain caused by my mom's actions finally took their toll. Or maybe Lori just discovered a love for cookies. I didn't know. And I did my best to recognize that Lori was on her own individual path in life, a path that wasn't going to necessarily be the same as mine.

Realizing Lori didn't want any part of my discoveries, I backed away slowly. Besides, I still had a lot of work to do on myself.

Having taken off 250 pounds just two years earlier, I was still armed with an arsenal of knowledge regarding healthy eating. And yet, I knew something about this time needed to be different. As I sat in my car, parked outside my apartment, downing two burgers, an order of fries, onion rings, two Sprites, and a milkshake, I realized that this was an "off" (the diet) moment. And that my dieting efforts had recently been about being "on" or "off."

I began to comprehend that for someone who used to weigh over 450 pounds (and could clearly get back up that high or *higher* again), there really could be no more "on" or "off." I realized I needed to think less in terms of "diet" and more in terms of "way of life."

I recommitted to following the basic tenants of my earlier "eating plan" (my new go-to words instead of diet), and I was now doing so with lots of flexibility. I knew I needed to take off 100 excess pounds and that would require some strict behavior. But I also knew that I could stick to that plan without the severe "on-off" mentality that had always been one of my catalysts for cheating in the past.

No, this didn't mean I would allow myself to eat Ethel M chocolates during the two months of the year they were appearing throughout our advertising agency like demonic gremlins. But it did mean that I would occasionally have something to eat that wasn't necessarily on my eating plan. And that was when I got it: I didn't have to be all "last-supper syndrome" about it and have more than a healthy portion of it.

When enjoying the occasional treat, I would remind myself that this wasn't the last time I'd be eating it and that I could have it, and enjoy it again, in the future.

A Typical Day on Gregg's SF Diet

BREAKFAST

½ of a Whole Grain Bagel

1 tbsp. All Natural Peanut Butter

1 small or medium Banana

Coffee

LUNCH

Lunch Salad

6 oz. of Broiled Chicken, chopped into chunks

2 cups fresh Cherry Tomatoes, sliced in half

Balsamic Vinegar and Fresh Ground Pepper

DINNER

6 oz. Swordfish Steak

(Seasoned with fresh Ground Pepper, Garlic Powder, and Balsamic Vinegar)

Organic Salad Greens

½ cup sliced Cherry Tomatoes

½ cup sliced Cucumber

EVENING SNACK

1 medium Fuji Apple

AND THROUGHOUT THE DAY

Lots and lots of water (room temperature)

(For a treat, I'd have Sparkling Water with meals)

Was everything perfect in my life as a result of the therapy? No. In fact, there were lots of imperfect things in my life. But with some clarity regarding my mom's actions being in the *past* and my actions affecting my *present*, I knew that with a little work and tough love I could get rid of those pesky 100 pounds once again. And, perhaps, once and for all.

I once again tried to focus more on why I wanted to be thin and healthy. I pulled out and dusted off my Me Book and got in touch with what I would gain from taking off the excess 100 pounds, rather than focusing on what I was giving up. I was again inspired by the pictures, articles, and other reminders as to why looking and feeling good was better than a cheeseburger or whatever.

I began exercising more regularly, having realized that I had been using my excuse of the long commute to and from work as to why I "didn't have time to work out."

This excuse of not being able to work out seemed especially true given that the closest gyms to my apartment were not open during hours that I needed them to be. But this is when I remembered that living in the Marina area of San Francisco meant that I could easily walk down to the Marina Green, which happened to be right on the bay, and power walk to my heart's content. I had copies of the music mixes from the aerobics classes I took in New Jersey, which I played as I strutted my stuff in circles around the green. I pumped my arms, I lifted my chest, I sucked in my stomach, and I worked out (walked out), daily.

Anytime I was able to make it to the gym before it closed, I would take an exercise class of some kind. Because it was usually later in the evening, a lot of times the only class offered was yoga. I had never taken any kind of yoga class before and was quite intimidated by the concept. But living in San Francisco, I'd heard that it was beneficial for all kinds of reasons, including mental health. So I decided to dip my big, clumsy toe into the yoga waters.

My first class felt a lot like doing Origami, where I was the piece of paper that got folded up in a rather complicated way. I didn't know what I was doing, but the instructor was kind and took her time with me. Before long I was, ahhh, heck. I was always clumsy when taking yoga and still am to this day. But I do love the concept of working out my inner body, organs, mental awareness, etc., along with my outer body to become leaner and more flexible. I found this to be a great addition to the cardio exercise I was getting from my power walks.

There I was working my body, mind, and spirit all at the same time. And the scale responded accordingly. The weight once again began to melt away. And soon I had more than just one pair of pants to wear to work.

At the same time, I did some inner work on my personality as well. No longer was I saying things to people that I thought might win them over. I tried to approach coworkers and potential friends with more authenticity. I didn't want to be my mother and tell people the story I thought they wanted to hear. Instead, I was real with myself and real with them. Never disrespectful, but real.

I realized a lot of this effort to communicate in a more authentic way would entail treating people like people and not like shiny, pretty objects. In my recent past, I saw that I had acted as if people like Linda were Barbie dolls of sorts, that is, things I wanted to add to my collection for face value, rather than real value. So I decided to change the way I approached people, including Linda, who I made a point of re-introducing myself to in a more authentic way.

Before long, Linda and I became good friends and we spent endless hours laughing as we worked together. In fact, there were times we laughed so hard that people would look at us and wonder what we were smoking. But we weren't smoking anything. We were just being real with one another. And that was cause not only for laugher, but for joy. An authentic joy I was experiencing perhaps for the first time in my life.

ANOTHER PERSPECTIVE
ON GREGG AT THIS TIME

By Linda Souders, Gregg's Coworker at the SF Agency

First let me say how flattered and delighted I am to be chosen as Poster Girl for the "pretty people" at the agency. However, my soul knows that any beauty Gregg saw in me was merely a reflection of his own magnificence being mirrored back to him.

I distinctly remember the moment I met Gregg. I was on the phone with the account executive assigned to his and my first project together. She said to me, "The copywriter will be Gregg McBride." His name echoed inside me like a sounding bell heralding the arrival of someone great.

When I phoned Gregg to introduce myself and inquire about carpooling to meet the client, I was met with a cool aloofness. I wasn't deterred by his reserve, being accustomed to guardedness in others, especially new acquaintances.

Gregg says I held him at arm's length in the beginning until he began to approach me more authentically. But honestly I kept most people at arm's length. I wasn't treating him any differently from anyone else. I think he simply saw it that way. As we all often do, we feel we are the only one. But truly, behavior is never singular. The way we treat one is the way we treat all. I, too, was cool and aloof and safe inside my closed clam shell. I am one of those people who don't warm easily. I had my own history and scars and baggage to protect.

Reading Gregg's account of how he felt during that time surprises me because he seemed to feel that he was the only one on the outside looking in. But I was feeling on the outside that whole time too. I believe many of us feel this way. We feel what Lily Tomlin so aptly captured when she said, "We are all in this alone, together." It's impossible to climb inside someone else's skin. Or to invite others into ours. The best we can do is extend compassion. Gregg got that. And did that.

What I remember most about our time together was Gregg's extraordinary sense of humor. I find the saying "laughter is the best medicine" to be completely accurate. Gregg's constant wit was the morphine drip that kept me going through the long, grueling, pressure-filled hours at the agency. Gregg was the bright spot—shining through the nine-to-five grind. He made life in the trenches bearable. His wit cut right through the uptight, PC, business air of pretension. He constantly had me giggling, doubled over in side-splitting laughter. Next to him I felt like a kid, rebellious and carefree.

I relished trips to Gregg's office downstairs. The objective was to collaborate on the copy and art we were creating for our clients, but the greater product was the uplifting of my spirit from our laughing together. I always went back to my office giddier, happier.

If there are past lives, I am certain Gregg and I know each other from before. He felt as comfortable to me as a brother. I gave him the nickname "Bifford," "Biffy" for short. I called myself Gabrielle. He was my twin. If our lives were a movie, he would be the one at the blue-blood family gathering, dressed in monogrammed ties and penny loafers, setting off fire crackers in the bushes next to the buffet table, constantly wreaking havoc. I snickered in delight as the uptight adults winced. In this life, we made a play of our time together. Few others got it, which brought us even closer. We shared a secret language that few others could understand.

Gregg did bring up his weight struggles with me, although always in his off-the-cuff, casual way. That refreshing candidness created a personal connection. Where other colleagues created distance through their guardedness, Gregg managed to remove the wedge between us. His ability to let down his guard and allow others to see him authentically was a breath of fresh air. It was intoxicating. I wanted to be around him. As he melted his armor, he made it possible for me to melt mine a bit too, and draw closer to him.

I loved spending time with Gregg because he has an elegance, a refinement to his character, and an air of royalty. Not a calculated or forced sense of appropriateness, but a graceful quality inherent to his being. I believe each of us finds kindred spirits along our life paths. People who resonate with us naturally. Gregg is that person for me.

CHAPTER NINE

the big skinny

With eight months of healthy eating behind me, along with healthy physical and mental exercising, I was once again seeing the results I wanted to see. The scale was registering around 185 pounds and I was fitting into clothes I hadn't been able to wear in over a year.

I wasn't in touch with my mother, and I didn't feel the need to be. She was living her life. I was living mine. I was an adult now and I didn't need her approval, not even her admission that I wasn't really adopted, in order to be me.

And yet, I was still suffering from a fat mentality.

Just as had happened when I lost the initial 250 pounds in New York, I was now left with a lot of saggy, baggy skin. My body may have only weighed in at around 185 pounds, but I still had enough skin to accommodate a 450-plus pound man.

Getting dressed was a chore, even when putting on so-called skinny clothes and wearing outfits that I bought at the Gap, Banana Republic, J. Crew, and other stores that had never catered to me at larger sizes. I had an average-size waist but I had to buy larger sizes in order to make room for the loose skin, which I would have to tuck into whatever I was wearing.

It made no difference that I was exercising four to five times a week, that I was eating healthy foods, or that I was doing yoga for my internal and mental health. I still had mounds and mounds of loose skin to contend with. And even after trying to conceal the masses of skin hanging from my chest, stomach, back, pelvis, and thighs, I would still have the appearance of "puffiness," no matter what I was wearing. This was very disheartening and took a lot of wind out of my sails.

As if to make matters worse, I was noticing another side effect of all of my loose skin. When walking quickly, like during my power walks on the Marina Green or when running or even dancing, I would notice a "swooshing" sound. It was as if someone was swishing water around a large fish tank. At first, I was as confused as anyone around me wondering where the sounds were coming from. Until I realized the "swooshing" was coming from me.

One Thanksgiving morning, I was watching the Macy's Thanksgiving Day Parade on television with some friends. At one point I decided that I needed to be silly and dance along with the performers on TV. So I jumped up and started moving to the music. Suddenly, my roommate Nik asked, "What's that sound?"

I stopped dancing. We all listened. The swooshing sound had stopped. I was as baffled as everyone else . . . until I started moving again and realized that the swooshing was the flaps of loose skin around my upper thighs moving to and fro as I danced along with the TV performers.

Before anyone else could notice the sound was coming from me, I made an excuse to leave the room and rushed to the bathroom. I shut the bathroom door and locked it. Now by myself, the sound of the swooshing echoed through my head, even though I remained frozen with embarrassment. No one mentioned the sound when I returned from the bathroom, but it was clear we all knew where the noises had been coming from. They were coming from me.

I made sure to move very slowly throughout the rest of the day. I'm sure I looked ridiculous, as if I were moving in slow motion. But I was mortified and didn't want to be identified with that swooshing sound again.

Later, I did some research into the loose skin phenomenon that plagues people who've taken off a lot of excess body weight. Like many, I had no idea this was a common ailment and thought I was the only one whose skin didn't somehow magically retract. I'd always thought that exercise would take care of the excess skin. But it did not.

It turns out that this is one of those topics to do with weight loss that not many people, not even the so-called experts, talk or write much about. But loose skin is an unavoidable problem when someone loses an enormous amount of excess body weight, like it or not.

I couldn't believe it. Here I'd spent most of my life trying to lose weight with the goal of being able to wear a bathing suit and not have people wonder if I was male or female because of my man boobs. But even after losing the weight, a hundred pounds of it more than once, I was more embarrassed than ever to take off my shirt.

Not only did I have saggy, baggy "moobs" (short for "man boobs" for those not in the know), but my body was also covered in stretch marks. The loose skin around my abdomen hung down over my penis so far that I had to lift it up when standing and urinating—to say nothing of the swooshing skin around my thighs and upper arms.

This was made worse by the fact that whenever I would sweat, I would get rashes on the areas where the loose skin was folded up whenever I was wearing clothes. I was going through more body powder than a baby wearing a diaper. And despite using powder, the rashes would still occur.

I thought of myself as a hideous freak, and there didn't seem to be anything I could do about it, other than to move slowly and buy stock in baby powder.

So move slowly I did for the next several months. I would never accept an invitation to go power walking with someone else, much less dancing unless it was at a club that played really loud music. And I made sure to wear long sleeves and long pants even on the warmest days.

Many times I wondered to myself why I'd even bothered losing the weight to begin with, or why I was trying to maintain the weight loss. At least when I weighed over 450 pounds I was "solid." Now, after taking off all the weight, I was still "bulge-y" when wearing clothes. I made sounds when I moved. And I was covered in sweat or rashes.

After about a year of living in virtual misery like this, I decided to seek out a surgeon to investigate what it would take to get rid of the excess skin once and for all. I soon found out that cosmetic (or "plastic") surgeons perform loose skin removal surgery. I'm not sure how I ended up choosing the surgeon I did. Truthfully, it was dumb luck since I didn't dare ask anyone I knew for a recommendation. I didn't want to tell them why I needed a plastic surgeon.

Much like my therapist, the plastic surgeon I ended up going to was gruff, to-the-point, and forthright. This turned out to be a good thing, mainly because he was honest about the costs that would be involved with skin removal surgery (insurance would not cover a cent of it) and the likely side effects of the surgery (like scarring). He showed me several "before" and "after" pictures, usually of breast reduction surgery, since he'd never before performed a skin reduction surgery on someone who had lost as much weight as I had.

The evidence in the "after" photographs showed that all surgical patients had scars where their excess breast skin or abdomen skin had been. In other words, they looked better, but certainly not perfect. Nor did they look "magazine appearance ready," which is something I'd always envisioned being when wanting to lose weight.

Well, turns out it didn't matter that there were going to be scars and other after-effects from the surgery, because I couldn't afford the surgery in the first place. The doctor explained that surgery of this nature would require a hospital stay, which meant I'd be looking at a total cost of around $20,000 or higher.

No way. No how.

I decided I needed to learn to live with the loose skin.

NAKED AMBITION

I thought perhaps I was making too big of a deal out of the loose skin. Maybe I saw it as much worse than it really was. After all, no one else had seen me naked in recent years. Actually, no one else had seen me in short sleeves, shorts, or even a bathing suit in recent years.

So when an agency business trip brought me out to New York City for some meetings, I took the opportunity to spend a little time with my friend Elizabeth. Having been close for years and years, I asked her if she would be willing to look at me naked. After she stopped laughing and realized I wasn't kidding, bless her heart, she said she would.

Thinking back, I should have sensed the hesitation in Elizabeth's agreement. I mean, we were never romantically involved. So for her to agree to take a good, long look at a naked man she wasn't intimately involved with really was an act of true friendship.

But even with this close to lifelong friend, I was terrified to disrobe. In the grand tradition of the Cowardly Lion, I made Elizabeth promise to keep her eyes shut until I'd completely undressed. I then clamped my eyes shut out of fear of seeing her reaction when I told her to open hers.

I kept my eyes shut as I spun in a slow circle so Elizabeth could check out all angles of my naked form, and I made her watch me bend over, which sent all my loose skin cascading in one direction like a tidal wave of Jell-O.

I'm happy to report that Elizabeth did not try and flee the room while my eyes were closed.

I quickly got dressed and then opened my eyes, anxious to see what kind of terrified look she had on her face after seeing me nude—stretch marks, loose skin, and all.

I'm not going to lie. There was an unsettled look on Elizabeth's face. But there was also a genuine sense of empathy, and an unspoken understanding of what I was going through.

She was very calm while she explained that some of what she saw was a little off-putting. But she was quick to point out that there were areas of her own body that she was embarrassed of as well, admitting that she, too, had stretch marks around her ample breasts. She then explained that anytime I got undressed, it would likely be with someone who cared about me and would, as a result, accept me.

"And when in doubt," Elizabeth joked, "Keep the lights dim."

Talk about a bonding experience. I still can't believe I subjected myself—not to mention Elizabeth—to that "viewing." But it was something I felt I needed to do at the time. And now? I was ready to do it with someone I cared about, romantically.

To say my unveiling with a potential paramour went well would be an overstatement. When I decided to take a chance with the then partner of my dreams, I didn't get naked right away. Instead, I accepted a pool date and decided I was going to wear my bathing suit proudly, not worrying about how my body looked.

Things seemed to go okay at the pool. After I summoned up enough nerve to take off my T-shirt, I was relieved when time didn't stop, the world didn't end, and my date didn't run screaming.

However, I later learned from a mutual friend that my pool date described my body as looking like a Shar Pei dog, the breed known for its flaps of skin that hang from its body.

Being compared to a Shar Pei dog was too much for me.

Instead of being mad at my date for describing me as such, or at the so-called friend who callously told me about it, I got angry at myself, as if there was something I could do about the loose skin all over my body. There wasn't. I couldn't afford the surgery and, even if I could, I would still be left with the scars and stretch marks.

I entered a deep depression after that. But instead of bingeing I began to emulate my semi-anorexic days in New York and ate less and less. And no matter how much "less" I ate, the loose skin situation only got worse. Thanks to my busy schedule and my four to five times a week exercise regimen, I soon realized that the eating less was adversely affecting my energy level. So that form of self-abuse didn't last very long. But the loose skin and its effects on my psyche were haunting me.

Then came the day I fit into a size thirty-five-inch waist at Banana Republic. Despite a lengthy time at around 185 pounds, which was my now average body weight, I hadn't quite accomplished that feat. But there I was, in the Banana Republic dressing room, zipping and buttoning up those thirty-five-inch waist pants without even holding my breath.

I assumed my best attempt at a supermodel pose and looked at myself in the mirror, marveling at my feat. For someone who used to struggle wearing a size sixty-inch waist, donning a size thirty-five-inch waist was a major accomplishment. And yet, when I turned to the side to do a little more marveling, there it was—the "puff" of fabric that jettisoned out from my upper groin area, the part of the pant that was stuffed with the loose skin hanging from my abdomen.

Standing in that particular dressing room on that particular day was my breaking point. I decided I was too young and had worked too hard to have to deal with this loose skin for the rest of my life.

Shar Pei dog my ass.

I called the plastic surgeon I'd met with earlier in the year. My question wasn't whether or not he would do the surgery, but whether or not his office accepted credit cards.

That's right. I didn't have a savings account at the time. And I wasn't making the kind of money from advertising to afford plastic surgery. But I did have a few credit cards that I wasn't using at all.

So I decided to put my skin reduction surgery on two different credit cards.

To this day I am grateful to the doctor and to his wife, who manages his office. Sensing my sincerity, knowing my determination, and being aware of my income situation, they helped keep the expenses and fees as low as possible. In fact, the greatest expense was going to be my overnight stay at the local hospital. The doctor warned me it would be key to keep that stay to one night, because those were fees that he could not control.

Even with all of this helpful information, I was not mentally prepared for the surgery itself. It turns out a lot of plastic surgeons' offices aren't always forthcoming about what the real recovery time will be immediately following (and weeks or months following) the surgery.

The weeks leading up to the surgery were frightening. I wasn't sure what to expect, or how much of the loose skin problem the surgery would fix. In order to keep expenses down they were going to do all of the surgery at one time. And even then, there would be areas of my body they wouldn't be able to "get to."

I was so nervous the night before I was scheduled to check into the hospital that I binged. Not parked in my car, but parked in my living room, eating most of a pizza while looking out of the bay window onto other rooftops populating the San Francisco Marina District. I wondered how much this surgery would affect my life—professionally, romantically, and otherwise.

Gregg's Night Before Skin Removal Surgery Binge

6 slices of Cheese Pizza

1 small bag of Potato Chips

1 giant Chocolate Chip Cookie

I also feared for my nipples. Why? The doctor had explained that removing the excess skin from my chest area would require completely removing my nipples and then stitching them back into place. He warned me that some people cannot feel their nipples, having no more sensitivity to touch, etc., after this type of surgery.

"But sometimes they can?" I asked.

"Sometimes," the doctor replied.

Damnit. I wanted to feel my nipples in the future. But I knew after my surgery that might no longer be the case.

GOING UNDER THE KNIFE

Reporting to the hospital before sunrise was nerve-racking. I felt like I had to confess that I had binged the night before, even though I had stopped eating before a certain time, as instructed. I wanted to tell them about my elaborate meal and find out if we should postpone the surgery for another time, after I had a little more time to take off a few more pounds. I was being very dramatic.

The doctor thought it was all very amusing, and his attitude calmed me. I was still giving him "last minute instructions," while an attendant administered general anesthesia and told me to count backward from ten.

I panicked. I'd seen way too many movies with scenes of surgery going wrong. I knew I'd get to "one" and they'd all look foolish once I did.

10 . . . 9 . . . 8 . . . My eyes blinked. But I was still awake.

I looked around, asking the nurse where the doctor was. I explained that I had to give him a few more mandates before the surgery. The nurse chuckled as I began to notice the tubes coming out of my arms, all leading up to bags full of different liquids that hung above me.

I had just been brought to. The seven-and-a-half hour surgery was complete.

That night at the hospital was quite uncomfortable. I had stitched up "wounds" all over my body—my chest, upper arms, abdomen/pelvis area, and upper thighs. There were several draining tubes in use. I was on morphine, so I didn't have a total sense of the pain, but I distinctly remember the feeling of areas of my body having been cut into pieces and reattached.

I didn't sleep much during the night. Nurses constantly checked on me, wanting to know if I had been able to use the bathroom. Apparently that was the goal. I had to be able to stand, move to the bathroom, with assistance, and "go" on my own before I would be released from the hospital. I needed to meet that goal, as there was no way I could afford a second or third night in that place.

At one point it was deemed "too long" since I'd urinated, and a nurse arrived to insert a catheter. Despite being on a morphine drip, I experienced every second of unrelenting pain from having that thing inserted. That god-awful, super-agonizing moment would become what Oprah calls an "aha moment."

For it was while the catheter was being administered that I decided I was going to leave my comfortable life working in advertising in San Francisco and move down to Los Angeles to pursue my true dream of screenwriting within the next year.

Yep. That was the moment that decision was made. And I can say, since the catheter was being inserted at the time, it was one of the most painful decisions I've ever made in my life.

The next morning, I had my doctor and a few of his colleagues gathered around me, checking my wounds. Some were still draining, but everything looked "good." The doctor explained that he removed over one and a half yards of skin from my body (over twelve pounds!). He considered the surgery a success and my wounds seemed to be healing well.

But now was the big test; could I urinate on my own?

Not wanting to pay for another night in the hospital, I rose from bed and took a very slow walk to the restroom. I managed to squeeze out a few drops of urine, which was good enough for the doctor. I was released from the hospital.

My roommate Nik was ready to drive me back to our apartment, but I could barely bend down enough to get in the car, much less handle the pain of the ride home on what seemed like the bumpiest road in Marin county. We made it only a mile or two before pulling over to the nearest motel, where we spent two nights as I recovered more fully. Nik was a champ—administering medicine, emptying the bedpan we'd been given by the hospital and even draining my tubes, all things a roommate should never be asked to do.

It was about that time that I realized the recovery period was going to be lengthier than I'd imagined. Since I was now working as a freelancer and no longer as a full-time employee at the advertising agency, I was able to stay home to recover. But I could barely move, much less walk or care for myself.

I wasn't allowed to shower for a couple of weeks and had to wear a tight-fitting spandex bodysuit that would "encourage" my skin to re-adhere to my body's frame, since it had been literally pulled away and then tightened during the surgery. The discomfort was unbearable, as was the inability to move.

I had no choice but to lie on my back, except for a few times a day when Nik would help me sit up in order to eat food he had prepared. I had him fix me very strict diet food at the time, knowing I wasn't getting any movement, let alone exercise, and that I was therefore expending far fewer calories than usual. Plus, the doctor had warned me not to gain *any* weight during the first six months, while the skin was still re-adhering itself to my body.

A Typical Day on Gregg's Post-Surgery Diet

BREAKFAST

1 cup Cold Cereal

1 cup Skim Milk

1 small Banana

Water

LUNCH

6 oz. Protein (usually Turkey cold cuts)

2 cups Lettuce/Tomatoes

Dressing

Balsamic Vinegar/Olive Oil/Dijon Mustard mix

AFTERNOON SNACK

1 piece of Fruit (usually an Apple)

DINNER

1 small can of Tuna fish

(Seasoned with Fresh Ground Pepper and Balsamic Vinegar)

½ cup sliced Cherry Tomatoes

½ cup sliced Cucumber

Twice a week I allowed myself to have a smoothie Nik would pick up from a local deli down the street. Those were frozen moments of heaven.

Just walking and going to the bathroom took every ounce of energy I had. Other than that I was laid out on my back, and, yes, there were resulting bedsores. At night I was only allowed to maintain one "sleeping" position—on my back—and I didn't even have the wherewithal to get up by myself to use the restroom. So I had to use a bedpan that Nik would empty after use. Those were truly some of the most painful days of my life, and just as bad for Nik, I'm sure.

Two weeks passed and I was finally approved to take a shower. I shuffled to the bathroom like a man in his nineties. I needed to learn how to walk again after being off my feet so long. The wounds and stitches covering my body severely inhibited most kinds of movement.

Getting out of the tight-clinging body suit was awful. At that point it was basically attached to both me and my wounds. It took over an hour to remove, after which Nik, quickly and thankfully, rushed it to the washing machine in our apartment building's basement.

Left alone in the bathroom, I positioned myself in front of a large mirror and finally got up the nerve to take a look at my body. I stared for several minutes, taking it all in. And then . . . I started to cry.

I looked like Frankenstein's Monster, stitched virtually from head to toe—even though one couldn't actually see the stitches since most of them were just underneath the incisions. The long "slit-style" wounds were plentiful, and each was red from irritation. My nipples, which I wasn't sure whether I could feel or not, were not on the same plane. One was headed north. The other was headed south. I cried more, wondering what I'd done to myself.

After a few more minutes I managed to take a painful step into the tub. Just stepping over the tub's edge caused agonizing pain. I had no range of motion. After getting into the tub, pulling the shower curtain closed, and turning on the water, I tried to lift my arms overhead so that the water could run under my arms. I couldn't even get my arms to shoulder level. They wouldn't lift. The wounds prevented me from doing so.

That "first shower" ordeal led to several panicked calls to my doctor. He was always calm and reassuring, even available after hours, telling me to give my body "time to adjust." I'd had no idea I would have to go through such a lengthy recovery phase. I'd thought perhaps I might not be able to drive for a couple days, but never that I wouldn't be able to walk for several weeks.

When going in for checkups, my doctor would always remind me that "we" never know how the human body will react to these kinds of surgeries. And that's true. But honestly, nothing could have prepared me for the six months of recovery I had to go through as a result of the skin removal surgery.

Granted, I'd had the surgery done in one fell swoop. But wouldn't most people have to do it that way? After all, who has the kind of budget, let alone the kind of time, to undergo such a life-inhibiting event?

Eventually, I didn't have to wear the spandex bodysuit anymore. That was a huge relief, though I felt very vulnerable when first venturing out into the world without having it on under my clothes.

Just getting up and down the stairs to and from my fourth floor apartment was a major feat and took a great deal of time, but I was determined to begin exercising again. At first I could only shuffle around the block one time, but soon I rediscovered my stamina and before too much longer I was shuffling around the Marina Green.

Eventually all movement returned. I could lift my arms over my head; I could power walk when exercising; and my nipples even returned to the same vicinity. No, my nipples aren't quite on the same plane. But I am happy to report that when I touch them, I can feel the touch.

Mission accomplished.

The only thing left to do was nominate my roommate Nik for sainthood for his devotion to my healing during that lengthy post-surgery process.

During a follow-up visit months later, I asked why plastic surgeons' offices aren't more upfront about what to really expect after undergoing plastic surgery. They explained that if people really knew what they were in for, they wouldn't be as willing to go through with it. And you know what? I have to agree.

I had no idea about the torture and torment that lay ahead of me prior to the surgery. Had I known—*really known*—I'm honestly not sure I would have gone through with it.

Now that most of my excess skin had been excised, there was still some major mental baggage that needed to be taken care of.

ANOTHER PERSPECTIVE
ON GREGG AT THIS TIME

By Nik Sklaroff, Gregg's Roommate in San Francisco

Few things in life are as painful as watching another person suffer and being unable to do anything to help him or her. Knowing the suffering is a matter of choice, not an accident or a tragedy, makes seeing such pain even more unbearable.

When Gregg made the choice to get surgery, I didn't understand why he felt the need for it and why he chose to put himself through the ordeal. I had little comprehension of what the surgery would involve and how arduous the recovery process would be. If the doctors didn't fully prepare Gregg for the ordeal he was about to endure, his friends were even more in dark about what the days and weeks after the surgery would be like.

It is probably good that I didn't know what would come. I was— still am—too squeamish to volunteer for a job involving bedpans, drainage tubes, dressing wounds, and the dreaded "suit." But watching the pain my friend endured summoned my compassion and ability to overcome the squeamishness. Somehow we muddled through those long, trying days.

To this day it is painful to recall the time it took to carefully remove the spandex suit, feeling afraid that the wounds and stitches would come loose, and that one false move might open up the wounds or set body parts asunder.

The day Gregg removed the suit for the first time and found that his nipples were at different heights on his chest was particularly trying. Here he had gone through years of weight loss and exercise and now the most physically painful surgery, only to discover that instead of improving his looks, he had come out, apparently, disfigured.

Over the next few weeks, after assurances from the surgeon, his body healed and his nipples returned to their intended positions, but without doubt that was the lowest point of his recovery. The great unveiling was marred by the horror of the first look at the results and the fear of lifelong disfigurement. He was crushed, and I really feared for him.

As someone who has struggled all his life with weight loss, too, I marvel at the courage and perseverance it took for Gregg to undertake not only the surgery, but also the whole ordeal—the early morning workouts, the foregone meals, and all the other sacrifices and pains he endured to achieve the weight loss that preceded the surgery.

For many of us, weight loss is a series of mini-victories, followed by inevitable relapses and defeats. Gregg summoned a courage and strength to make it through those low points to continue in just one direction in order to meet his goal of achieving a "normal" weight.

I got to see and experience first-hand the physical pain that this transformation entailed. Little did I realize the real suffering, the real scars, were the ones that preceded the surgery. The wounds inflicted by insensitive comments. The rejections. It is based on this new understanding that it now makes sense why someone would voluntarily go through the surgery and such physical pain to heal the emotional wounds that preceded it.

AGE	WEIGHT
31	175 lbs.
Today	175 lbs.
I no longer weigh myself regularly!	

PART III

after

CHAPTER TEN

new and improved

For someone who never considered himself a "boob man," I was spending a lot of time staring at my chest. My nipples were still in flux. One day they would seem to be on more of an even plane. The next, they would be headed in two different directions. I was horrified and still wondered if I'd done the right thing by having the surgery.

But then I'd see that despite the scars there was no more excess skin hanging from my chest. My man boobs and their "sacks" were gone. Sure, the stretch marks were still there. And there was no way of telling how well the scars would heal over time. But for the first time since first grade I had a male chest. I decided this was a major accomplishment, regardless of which way my nipples were headed.

I did resent the scars and the stretch marks. I likened them to a prison tattoo that would forever testify to the fact that I used to be morbidly obese. There would be no hiding it, no matter what size clothing I was wearing. But yet, even with the remaining scars and stretch marks, something more began to happen, visually.

There was some slight muscle definition developing in my chest area. I could see the results of doing pushups after my power walking sessions. I couldn't believe it. Were it not for the scars, the stretch marks, and the wayward nipples, I would have taken a picture for all to see. Instead, this modest, newfound muscle definition was my quiet little secret, albeit an exciting one.

Needless to say, this development encouraged my working out, to the point that I began to research and develop my own weight-lifting routines. I wasn't interested in morphing into a bodybuilder, but I was excited to see some physical results from my workouts. Before too long, I saw some definition in my stomach area as well. There was no visible four-, six-, or eight-pack; but there was some definition. You could look at my stomach and see some of the muscles under the skin. This, my friends, felt like a true milestone.

As I ramped up my workouts, more people started to take notice. The feedback from friends and colleagues wasn't so much about how I looked, as it was about how I moved. Lots of people told me that since the excess skin was cut away, I carried myself much differently. The bulk of the comments I received was that I appeared "lighter" and "less bogged down."

This resulted in my working more on my posture in order to communicate a loftier self-esteem. It wasn't the easiest thing. Besides, being a writer and therefore permanently hunched over a laptop trying to think of a good adjective to pair with a certain blouse or dog toy, I found that standing up straight was made more difficult by the surgery itself. It was like I had been tightened up and couldn't stretch back out. When I stood up straight, I could feel my skin, and even my incisions, straining. But no matter, I was committed to reaching higher—both figuratively and literally—and ultimately I was truly feeling the positive results of the surgery.

This was all very good news, because there were still moments when I questioned whether or not the surgery was worth it. Besides the grueling six-month recovery period and the significant scar tissue still forming on my body, I was also paying off the credit cards I'd used to fund the surgery and my hospital stay.

What's more, the scars seemed to be getting worse. Initially, the two sides of my skin—where there had been an incision to cut away skin in between—were just lined up next to one another, with most of the dissolvable stitches placed *under* the skin. But as time went on the scar tissue became more dimensional, even though I was keeping the scars out of the sunlight as instructed and putting my surgeon-prescribed ointment on them daily.

My doctor had warned me, "You never know how skin is going to react to being cut." And my skin was definitely *reacting*.

I was wearing smaller-sized clothes and had settled at a weight of around 175 pounds. I was finally an "after" as opposed to a "before." And yet, unlike the airbrushed or photo-shopped images we see in the media and online, I was the real-life version of an "after."

Scars.

Stretch marks.

And even some remaining saggy skin in places like my lower back, where my doctor wasn't able to reach during the single surgery.

Interesting side note: The doctor's wife told me the likely reason I didn't have to have any surgery to remove loose skin from my face or neck, two areas where there was no discernable loose skin, was probably because I incorporated animal protein into my diet while losing all the weight. Who knew?

I wanted to be grateful for all the changes that had and were taking place with my body. But I still felt ugly due to the scars and stretch marks. As mentioned before, I'd always dreamed of being "magazine ready" after losing the weight.

I wasn't.

I realize now that my ego was being exceptionally unreasonable. I share this egotistical side of myself in order to inform in a way that many so-called diet programs do not: We will always be a work in progress. No matter what side of the scale we are (or were) on.

The fact is that when I looked in a mirror, even with some definition around my chest and stomach, I was still seeing a fat person. I hated how I looked and found endless flaws to point out to myself while standing naked in the bathroom. My self-loathing seemed almost worse now than it had been when I weighed over 450 pounds.

What I had yet to connect with is that even though I'd gotten rid of the excess physical weight, I was still carrying around the mental weight. But that wasn't a lesson I was willing to embrace just yet.

This in turn led to some dangerous eating—in that I was eating very little for a certain time period post-surgery. I must have thought that if I ate less, the scars would become less noticeable, my stretch marks would fade, and the remnants of saggy skin would disappear overnight.

A Typical Day on Gregg's Post-Skin Removal Diet

BREAKFAST

½ of a Whole Grain Bagel

1 small or medium Banana

Coffee with Skim Milk and Artificial Sweetener

LUNCH

6 oz. Turkey Burger

Sliced Tomato

AFTERNOON SNACK

1 large Café Mocha (made with Skim Milk)

DINNER (IF ANY)

1 piece of Fruit (usually an Apple)

AND THROUGHOUT THE DAY

More Coffee with Skim Milk and Artificial Sweetener

What really happened as a result of that reckless eating was the opposite of what I'd hoped for. My skin got pastier, which showed off the scars and stretch marks even more; my energy decreased and even some of my newfound definition around my chest and abdomen disappeared. All because I wasn't consuming enough nutrients to sustain the muscle definition or any aspect of health.

Why was I torturing my body with such poor eating habits? Especially after all the research I'd done in regard to nutrition and being healthy? Those were questions I wouldn't have been able to answer at the time.

ROMANTICALLY CHALLENGED

There was one notion that would sometimes distract me from the self-loathing. I was ready to have Cupid shoot a few arrows my way. Though I was beating myself up mentally with negative self-talk and physically with poor eating habits, I was anxious to dip my toe back into the dating pool.

I still heard echoes of "his body reminds me of a Shar Pei dog" in my head, but the ever-hopeful romantic in me was sure that true love or, at least, true lust was waiting for me here, on the other side of excess skin removal surgery.

After a few awful first dates—on which I would still always fall in love after about five minutes, then be "heartbroken" when no second dates were granted—I had met someone I thought I might end up in bed with. The prospect of that was very exciting for someone who used to weigh over 450 pounds and who at one time paid a "professional" for an hour of simple cuddling.

I had a hunch my next date could lead to some real-life hanky panky. I was both thrilled and panicky. Thrilled for obvious reasons. Panicky for . . . well, perhaps just as obvious reasons.

I didn't verbalize my angst about my post-surgery body to many people, but I knew there was one person I could talk to: my dear friend Elizabeth who I had subjected my naked body to when it was still covered in loose skin. Ever the champ, Elizabeth listened intently while I explained to her that the person I was dating had no idea I used to be overweight, nor that I'd had one-and-a-half yards of excess skin cut away from my body about eight months earlier, leaving a plethora of scars.

After much debate, Elizabeth and I decided it was better not to say anything to my date beforehand and that, should the questions about the scars come up once I was undressed and in bed, that would be when I should provide a *"Reader's Digest* version" of the surgery details.

Okay. Good. Have the plan.

I had been right about this next date night. Dinner led to making out, which led to the bedroom. While the lamp next to the bed was a little too bright for my liking, I bravely started removing clothes, just as my date did. I was terrified. But I was also determined to get through this and to show off my new body with pride.

The shock and distaste in my date's eyes was evident from the get-go. And if it hadn't been, the statement from my date that "I feel sick. I think I need to cut this short," certainly revealed it.

I quickly dressed and fled the apartment, not sure what to think. I knew that somehow this debacle must have been my fault. But there seemed to be too many potential reasons to focus in on just one alone. So I scurried away from the light like any reasonable outcast would do.

The next morning I called Elizabeth and told her what had happened. She concluded, "Maybe you should have explained the scars *before* the unveiling."

Ya think?!

Ever the optimist and knowing how much I'd been looking forward to that encounter, Elizabeth encouraged me to call my date later in the day to check in. So I manned up and did just that. And, to my surprise, the call was answered.

"You weren't really sick, were you?" I asked.

"I was sick to my stomach, yes."

"Sick to your stomach? Why? Because I have a few scars?" I asked.

"You have scars covering your entire body. You should have told me."

"Should have told you what?" I pleaded. "About my surgery?"

"Yes. Anyone who has undergone a sex change shouldn't assume that people are going to be okay with it. There's no way I want to be physical with someone who used to be a girl."

Um . . . come again?!

Yup. That's right. Because I had significant scars around each nipple, in the vicinity of my chest, at my belly button, and right above my groin, it was assumed I had undergone a sex change and had breasts and a vagina removed and a fake penis put into place.

I tried to explain what my surgery was *really* about, but it was falling on deaf ears. Eventually I hung up the phone and never called back.

Elizabeth chalked all this up to "live and learn."

I, on the other hand, was convinced that I had just missed out on making mad, passionate love to the person who was destined to be the love of my life, and I was sure this had been my *very last chance* at romance and that I would now be alone, romantically speaking, for the rest of my days.

I really did think that belief was true, mainly because I wasn't going to take off my clothes for anyone ever again. In fact, at that moment, I committed to not looking into mirrors when undressing in the bathroom for the foreseeable future. My body was dead to me. And I was more ashamed of it than ever.

What I should have done is given myself a quick kick in the butt in regard to my ego's quest for perfection. Most of my freelance advertising work was now as an art and photo director, which meant I designed fashion catalogs, directing photographers and models on set. One thing I quickly learned about working with professional catalog models is that no matter how gorgeous they appear, they all have their issues, just like the rest of us. I worked with certain girls (I'm not being sexist—that's the term used on the set), who would know what kind of light flattered them (diffused) and what kind of light did not (direct sunlight). May the Lord help you if you or your photographer placed them in unflattering light. Same was true for unflattering clothing. Even if it meant giving up the shot to another model, these pros wouldn't be caught dead in clothing that showed them off in a way that wasn't flattering.

I share this because it's good news for all of us. Even professional models worry about their weight and their appearance.

Most of the models I worked with were hyper-intelligent. My explanation for this is that they are used to being treated as *objects* from an early age, so they learn to overcompensate in the smarts department in order to be taken seriously.

That was more good news as far as I was concerned, because many of the models I regularly worked with were extremely knowledgeable about health and nutrition.

Despite the fashion industry's reputation for bulimia and other eating disorders, many models in fact know they cannot eat in unhealthy ways and expect to keep working. Sure, they have to maintain a certain weight in order to wear and look good in clothes. But they also know that their skin tone needs to look healthy, their hair needs to be vibrant, and their mood needs to be level if they really want a full-time career.

So when I say that "models saved my life," I'm not being silly.

Over the years I had learned the tenets of healthy eating and managed to stay on a diet long enough to lose large amounts of weight, yet I had never really embraced making those habits a part of my everyday lifestyle. I still had a mentality of either being "on" or "off" where healthy eating was concerned.

The nasty "off" habit usually occurred on weekends, when I wouldn't be on any kind of diet at all starting on Friday and would eat anything I wanted through Sunday night, to the point of going to bed in pain. I would then re-start my healthy eating on a Monday, in a mad quest to lose the weight (water or otherwise) that I'd gained by overeating over the weekend.

One model I was excited to work with was Ulli Steinmeier. Ulli is a tall drink of water who hails from Germany. During the height of her modeling career, she was working alongside Cindy Crawford and other fashion world notables. I worked hard to land Ulli for the women's fashion catalog I was working on at the time. She didn't always agree to do catalogs, which many high-end fashion models considered "beneath them." But lucky for me, Ulli was willing to give it a try and, according to her agent, if she liked the vibe on set, would commit to the entire project.

When I first met Ulli, I fell into my old "trying too hard to please" mode, mimicking my mommy dearest by trying to be the person I *thought* Ulli would be interested in, as opposed to just being myself. Ulli smiled politely and nodded. But not much else.

One day we were alone in the makeup trailer and Ulli looked at me and said, in her sexy European accent, "Why don't you just drop the bullshit and be yourself?"

I was able to see the expression on my face in the large makeup trailer mirrors. I was completely dumbstruck. I looked like a jerk. Because I was once again acting like a jerk. My old habits of not being my authentic self were still lurking in the background. I realized I was participating in behavior that I abhorred—asking people questions without really listening to or caring about their answers, gossiping about others behind their backs, and pretending to know everything (when, really, I knew *nothing*).

Instead of getting defensive, bad mouthing Ulli, or heading directly to the craft services table to eat an entire plate of Fat Free Fig Newtons, I tried to take Ulli's advice to heart and worked to drop the

BS. Ulli's direct nature was the kick in the butt I had been in need of for some time. And you know what? It hurt so good.

I'm happy to say that once I dropped the BS with Ulli, I was more open to embracing the authentic people around me (on set and otherwise). This turned out to be a great thing since Ulli was very wise when it came to nutrition and exercise, as well as self-esteem. In fact, when she retired from modeling, she became a personal trainer and nutrition expert for geriatric patients in order to help them achieve a better quality of living.

Encouraged by Ulli and several other Southern California-based friends I'd met while on photo shoots in Los Angeles, I decided that now was the time to follow through on the promise I'd made to myself when the catheter was inserted and move to LA. I knew that pursuing my dream of screenwriting required me to live in Hollywood. And so I bid adieu to the Bay Area.

Though I had several friends in Los Angeles (including Ulli), relocating to that city was a frightening experience. Leaving San Francisco, where I was consistently getting a lot of work for my freelance advertising business, was a big leap. In Los Angeles, the business was all about show. There weren't a lot of catalogs being shot or even designed in LA, so I didn't have a great source of income while I toiled away trying to sell my first screenplay.

Surface dwelling Gregg didn't know to be bothered by those financial challenges though. While LA was new and "scary," I was only too happy to bail on whatever script I was working on in order to "do lunch" (or coffee, cocktails, or dinner) with my model friends.

The difference between my model friends and me was that they did have work from time to time—so they could pay their bills. But I had decided I'd be making a fortune on my first script sale (whenever that would be), so I could just "charge it" between now and then.

To make matters worse, unlike a few friends like Ulli who let me know when I was bordering on BS territory, a lot of people in LA welcomed another surface dweller. Who has time for true emotions and being real? This was Hollywood, and life here was a party. Or at least that's the hype I was buying into.

This was further complicated by me feeling like I might actually be one of the pretty people myself. No one knew I used to weigh over 450 pounds. They didn't even know that I'd had surgery to have a yard-and-a-half of excess skin removed (and I was never going to get undressed to let them know it either). So to my new LA "friends," I was just this hotshot creative guy from the Bay Area who wanted to be a screenwriter.

Welcome to the club.

Walking around LA was a trip. Strangers would approach me on the street to ask if I'd had plastic surgery. The first time that happened I was horrified, wondering who gave away my secret that I'd had excess skin removal surgery over a year ago. I was then relieved to find out that these strangers were (usually) admiring my nose, and they said so hoping that it had been "done" by a local plastic surgeon they could go to as well.

"Who did your nose?" they would ask.

I wanted to answer, "My mom's gene pool, but she'd never admit to it."

My self-esteem began to inflate after a few of those encounters— for all the wrong reasons. Needless to say, I wasn't hanging out with Ulli much at that time. Her bullshit sensor would have been worn out, at least in regard to my diet.

A Typical Day on Gregg's Initial Los Angeles Diet

BREAKFAST

(Usually slept through it)

LUNCH

Large Ice Blended or Vanilla Latte

1 low-fat Breakfast Muffin

AFTERNOON SNACK

Large Vanilla Latte (I was addicted at that point)

Piece of Fruit (usually a Banana)

DINNER

Cosmopolitan (Cocktail)

A few Chicken Wings (or other kind of appetizer-y food)

Dipping Sauce

AND THROUGHOUT THE DAY

More Coffee with Skim Milk and Artificial Sweetener

NIGHTTIME

Several Cocktails

WHEN RETURNING HOME (LATE AT NIGHT)

Several mouthfuls of Whatever was in the cabinets or refrigerator

I was as much of an idiot socially as I was nutrition-wise at that time. I fell back into some of my mother's "say whatever it takes to please anyone around you" mentality, operating along the brain patterns of a fat kid in the high school cafeteria: *I'll do anything to be popular*. Being "liked" by the Hollywood elite was validation for me (sad, but true).

This led to all sorts of misadventures I'm lucky didn't end any worse than they did. I might as well have been some yokel off the turnip truck in regard to not knowing what I was getting myself into.

LA was *all* about the nightlife. This meant sleeping late, then donning dark sunglasses and meeting someone late in the morning at The Coffee Bean and Tea Leaf for a Vanilla Latte or an Ice Blended. In LA we drink our calories. We don't eat them.

Next came the shopping. And I was all too good at this part of the day. After all, I had my "new" svelte, excess-skin-free body to outfit. I was determined to shop till I dropped—or until my credit score did.

Would I like to open a store credit card account? Why, yes, I would.

Next, after meeting for cocktails and a "light bite" (limited to two or three mouthfuls at the most), it was time to go home, take a catnap, get dressed, and then hit the clubs.

Did I mention the non-store credit cards necessary to keep up this aspect of the LA lifestyle?

Once in the nightclubs, I felt more like the fat kid in the high school cafeteria than any other time during the day. Although a big fan of music, I was not comfortable with myself on dance floors in LA, and I wasn't sure what kind of "lean against the wall" or "sit perched at a booth" position to take when not on the dance floor.

I hate to refer to myself as a cow, but that's what I was. I was being herded from here to there. At the time I thought I was living the dream. Here I was in Hollywood, partying with the beautiful people.

If only the people who knew me in high school as "foxy for a fat kid" could see me now.

Yeah. That's right. I was living my life trying to please not only people who weren't in my life anymore, but people who surely didn't care what I was doing or who I was doing it with.

My crowning achievement was making it into the VIP section of whatever nightclub I happened to be at. If I was with a group of "friends" that was within ten feet of a celebrity, I felt validated. I realize now I was so caught up in what I thought was validation for myself as a human being that I didn't realize how truly ignorant I had become. I was participating in everything that didn't matter and thought I was somebody because of it (when nothing could have been further from the truth).

DRUGS NOT HUGS

One night, while in the VIP section with a few "friends" I barely knew, I was told, "The party's moving." Being an obedient bovine, I was herded out of the club, where I was told to leave my car with the valet because this "big time producer" wanted us all to drive with him to his house in the valley.

"A big time producer (who I'd never met before that moment)? Okay."

Yokel. Turnip truck. Me.

While crammed into the backseat of a late model BMW with a bunch of other people, speeding down some unknown highway, I began to sense that everyone in the car had ingested some kind of a drug. Everyone's mood was just a little too good, a little too "revved up."

This was confirmed when a Quiet Riot song began to play over the car's stereo system and everyone started singing at the top of their lungs. Although a ham at heart, I wasn't familiar with hard rock. But I was too chicken to ask if they had any Hilary Duff on their playlist.

As the volume of the "singing" increased, so did the speed of the car. We were weaving in and out of traffic going at breakneck speeds. I wasn't as worried about being pulled over by cops as much as I was about ending up in a multi-vehicle accident. But even fearing for my life, I was still more afraid of what other people would think of me, so it was with great covert action that I reached down and fumbled around for a seatbelt, trying to put it on without being too obvious.

We ended up arriving at the "big time producer's" house safely. The grounds were quite expansive and everyone there, including people spilling out of a few other cars, seemed to know one another. Everyone but me, who only knew my friend I'd gone to the club with. Once inside, the hard rock began to play again as the producer pulled out a giant set of bongos and began playing them.

Everyone there seemed to be hitting an all-time high, which is when I noticed the plates, many plates, strewn all around the room with a pile of white, powdery substance on each one of them.

Up to then, the only powdery substance I was really familiar with was the kind that helped me avoid rashes when I had yards of excess skin to deal with. But this white, powdery substance was something entirely different.

Congratulations, Gregg. You've really arrived. You're at your first coke party.

Finally reaching the "freak out point," I retreated to the nearest bathroom, where I searched and searched for cell phone signal before being able to dial my friend Michele, whom I begged to come and pick me up. Even though it was 3:30 in the morning, Michele was willing to come and get me. Only she needed to know where I was.

Crap. Details.

I left the bathroom, managed to find the one person I knew, and told him my friend Michele, whom he also knew, was having an emergency and needed to come over. He was high enough on coke to give her the address without any questions.

When Michele arrived, she came in and sat next to me on the couch. Our mutual friend immediately grabbed a plate full of white powder and offered it to Michele. I jumped up and exclaimed, "We really need to get going. Michele has an emergency."

Everyone in the room quieted down and showed concern as Michele's and my mutual friend asked, "Oh, my god, Michele . . . What's the emergency?"

Being the crappiest friend ever (and the would-be screenwriter), I chimed in, "Yeah, Michele? What's the emergency?" She turned to look at me with mouth agape and then at our mutual friend and then back at me. Michele mumbled something about her boyfriend, a fight, and needing a place to stay.

After convincing the "big time producer" that we didn't want to stay at his home, Michele and I left, escaping the confines of the Valley and my very first (and only) coke party.

I was really handling LA well.

A few other social snafus and some blond highlights later, I got hit with enough credit card bills to give me pause. Only I was less concerned about the money and more concerned at how absentmindedly I was living my life.

Here I was in Los Angeles, a city I had dreamed of living and working in my entire life, and I was taking reckless physical and financial risks all because of a quest to be loved and accepted by those I perceived as beautiful. How had my self-worth become the equivalent of a picture in a catalog? And a small, insignificant picture at that? What had happened to me?

It didn't matter that I'd achieved the major feat of getting rid of over 250 pounds. It didn't matter that I'd overcome some insurmountable odds of childhood abuse and survived. It didn't matter that I had "real people" like Ulli in my life. I was still desperate. I was still insecure. I was once again morphing back into the person I swore I never wanted to be—my mother.

It didn't matter that the scale said I weighed around 175 pounds. I was carrying around more weight than ever.

ANOTHER PERSPECTIVE ON GREGG AT THIS TIME

By Ulli Steinmeier, One of Gregg's Fashion Model Associates

I think I like Gregg's definition of "supermodel" better than my own. When Gregg calls just about everyone he meets a supermodel, he does so to motivate them into realizing that they are the "shit" and can accomplish anything they set out to do—that there's no one better than them. And this is a definition I applaud.

I, however, know a different side to the term supermodel, having been a professional model (an oxymoron if ever I've heard one) for over twenty years.

I walked all those runways in Paris, Milan, New York, and practically everywhere else. Because of this I encountered "real life" supermodels, and just working models in general, who had only one diet they would go on to keep their ignorantly thin figures—a diet of cocaine, cigarettes, coffee, and champagne.

I was raised near a farm by parents who believed in wholesome nutrition (natural grains, lots of fresh vegetables, etc.), and so I learned the tenets of eating "right" at an early age. Even though I was offered a line of cocaine almost daily, and sometimes hourly, while as a "working girl," I never partook. I just didn't like the way it made me feel. You see, I learned that "how you feel" is the way you know whether or not you're eating right, and whether or not you're maintaining a healthy lifestyle.

By the time I met and started working for Gregg, I'd seen it all. So perhaps that's why I had the audacity to ask him to drop the bullshit. Walking onto the set of the catalog we were shooting, I was expecting nothing but another truckload of self-professed fashionistas, which usually included the crews behind the cameras, as well.

Even back in the day, everyone used tricks to make us models look nothing like we do in real life, both with our overly made-up faces (whether it looked like we had on makeup or not) and the portrayal of our unrealistically thin bodies. Before Photoshop there were other ways of deceiving the viewing public and of making them feel somehow inadequate. I assumed Gregg was just another engineer in that game of deception.

Upon closer examination, I realized Gregg was caught up in the glitz and smoke and mirrors just like the rest of us were. When someone first gets involved in the world of fashion, he or she usually can't help being seduced by the phony images and ego-boosters that the business offers. It's a pretend-world run by pretend-people. That doesn't mean I regret my years of modeling, but I don't regret getting out of the business either.

Today, I work as a trainer for geriatric patients who seek to increase their mobility and gain back a quality of life that might otherwise be eluding them. This kind of physical work is deeply satisfying. I suppose that's one of the reasons Gregg and I have not only kept in touch over the years, but have also gotten closer.

When I first met Gregg he may have seemed a bit vapid, having been enticed by the seductive world of fashion. But I've had the pleasure of seeing him evolve over the years into someone who truly knows and shows compassion. I love that today Gregg not only embraces his past (scars and all), but that he also shares it openly with others. He has gone through an incredible transformation, as much on the inside as on the outside, and the hard lessons he's learned are ones we can all benefit from.

CHAPTER ELEVEN

hollywood and *mine*

My excuses had all but run out.

For most of my life, I had blamed my excessive weight for not making friends, not finding work, not falling in love, and for anything else I wasn't achieving instantly. After the weight loss, I blamed loose skin and permanent stretch marks. After the loose skin was removed, I blamed the scars. And now? Despite the progress I'd made earlier with the therapist, I was still blaming my parents' abuse whenever necessary or convenient.

Pointing the finger came easily, as did being the self-proclaimed victim.

Here I was in Los Angeles, living my dream on the adventure ride called "life." And yet I thought I was miserable. I always kept my sense of humor and shared a lot of laughs along the way, but my cycles of self-abuse were once again rearing their ugly heads.

For example, I still wasn't eating right to maintain my weight loss, something that seemed even more important now that I lived in Hollywood.

A Typical Day on Gregg's Initial Hollywood Life Diet

BREAKFAST

Coffee with Cream and Sugar

LUNCH

Turkey Burger with only ½ Bun

Small Fruit Salad

AFTERNOON SNACK

Large Ice Blended or Vanilla Latte

DINNER

Giant bowl of Mixed Greens Salad (Enough to feed four)

With Dressing (Balsamic Vinegar, Dijon Mustard, very little Olive Oil mix)

Giant bowl of Chopped Fruit (usually Watermelon, also enough to feed four)

AND THROUGHOUT THE DAY

More Coffee with Skim Milk and Artificial Sweetener

While it was now with "healthier" foods, I was still often eating to excess, to the point of feeling stuffed on most days. This would result in poor nutrition and low energy, both of which I continued to mask through avid coffee consumption. Caffeine was my fuel of choice. Only I didn't want to admit the addiction to myself.

What I also didn't want to admit was that while I loathed her behavior, I was again living life in a way that was similar to my mother's modus operandi. I wasn't telling people I was a French princess with an adopted a child or two, but I would bend the truth every now and then. My lies were never overt. But if someone assumed something and I thought it might help my cause, I wouldn't correct him or her.

I was aghast that LA seemed to be full of surface dwellers, even though at the time I could have been accused of being the same. Everyone was caught up not only in finding out if you worked out, but where you worked out and who your instructors were. If you weren't paying thirty dollars plus for each exercise class, you weren't going to the right places or sweating with the right people.

I remember when first moving to LA, my friend Stephanie encouraged me to take classes with Bob Harper, notable for his appearances on the NBC television show, *The Biggest Loser*. To say Bob's exercise classes were intense would be an understatement. And everyone in those classes was there to be seen and to "work the room" before and after class. If you didn't know Bob's intricately choreographed aerobic routine, whether it was your first or your 100th class, Lord help you.

Dancing was never one of my strong suits. One time in Bob's class we were doing an intense aerobic routine using stairs. At one point (during a shift-step-cross-change or something like that), I tripped and fell down near my step. I looked to my friend Stephanie, who continued the routine with the rest of the class. She refused to look at me. And no one in the class—*no one*—checked to see if I'd broken a leg or twisted an ankle. I was Bob Harper roadkill. But I wasn't stupid. I quickly rose, composed myself, and got back into the routine, even though I could feel pain in my right foot. I was not staying down.

The same surface dwelling intensity applied to the rest of my daily routines in Los Angeles. I always joked that here you had to dress well twenty-four-seven, because people in LA get dressed up to take out the garbage. Oh, they might look like they're in their sweatpants. But you can bet those are $140.00 Juicy Coutures and not your every day, run-of-the-mill Gap sweats.

And only in the world of show business would it be just as important for writers and other professionals who work behind the cameras to look as good as the actors and actresses appearing in front of them. The only people in this business who seemed to be sporting any kind of beer belly were those who worked on movie set crews. And I'm pretty sure being part of their respective unions, they had a clause in their contracts that allowed for a little extra weight. But for the rest of us? We had to look as fit as our movie star counterparts.

My mom would have loved this seemingly vapid world where just about everything is pretend. And being her offspring, even though she wouldn't admit I was her offspring, I seemed to be fitting right in—well, except for that one time in Bob Harper's workout class.

SCREEN TIME

After my first official cocaine party, I decided I needed to hunker down in regard to my writing goals. After all, I did move down to Hollywood with the purpose of no longer just writing screenplays on the side, but actually selling a few. Besides that, I was running out of money from all of those LA lunches. Even my four times a day coffee habit was starting to add up, cost-wise.

I had a few scripts under my belt, and one of them finally started to gain some traction. It was an action movie called *Epicenter*. It was set in San Francisco and had lots of fun elements, which included a major earthquake at its core as well as a major subplot involving the crime world.

As a kid, I'd watched disaster movies on an endless loop. So I was thrilled when I found out that a studio not only wanted to buy my script, but actually put it into production. I would later learn that although you can sell a number of projects in Hollywood, actually getting them made is a completely different story.

I was initially put off by the fact that the studio in question was one that many would consider a B-movie company, meaning *Epicenter* was not going to be an A-list production. When writing the script, I'd imagined Jennifer Lopez playing the female lead (a tough cop with a young daughter who puts everything on the line).

Imagine my surprise when the B-movie company executives called me and told me they were really excited about casting Traci Lords (yes, the former porn actress) as the female lead. I learned that since she was once again trying to revive her professional career, she would be billed as Traci Elizabeth Lords.

In addition, they'd cast Gary Daniels (an international kickboxing champion) as the male lead, who would be playing the role of a banker. When the movie eventually had its Los Angeles premiere, I saw that the producers misspelled my name as "Greg McBride"—missing G—in the credits. Such is Hollywood!

But still, I was excited that my first feature was being made. I had to do a quick rewrite, the producers wanted the action to start in San Francisco but to have the big earthquake set piece actually occur in Los Angeles, but then production got underway.

Filming kicked off in Vancouver for the pre-earthquake sequences and then moved to an abandoned city in Romania for the post-earthquake scenes. I wasn't able to visit either of the sets because I had landed a staff writing job on the MTV show *Undressed* (a long-running drama on MTV airing after 11:00 p.m. that my friend Drew, a TV development VP, referred to as "a porn movie without the sex").

Yes, sex did have a lot to do with the stories we wrote about on *Undressed*. The title of the show wasn't *Fully Clothed* after all. The show focused on three different age groups as it told three different stories about high school-, college-, and post-college-aged characters.

It was while working on *Undressed* that I hit onto something big. Sure, *Epicenter* was a lot of fun to write. But I wanted to get to the hearts of some of the characters I created for *Undressed*, and to touch the hearts of viewers. I decided the best way to do this was to write about what I knew—being fat.

I decided I was going to get a fat girl's story onto a show that aired on a channel known for featuring only the sexy, alluring, and beautiful.

But pitching ideas for stories to *Undressed* executive producer and noted filmmaker Roland Joffé was a challenge. For one, Mr. Joffé seemed to respond more to ideas coming from female members of the writing staff rather than the males. But I wasn't about to let that stop me. So I had my friend Lizzy pitch my idea for me, knowing she would be fine with my claiming and writing it after its approval.

Sweetheart's Dance became a multi-episode story on *Undressed*, one that featured a female lead named Bonnie, an overweight high school student who not only ends up clashing with her school's would-be homecoming queen, but also ends up romantically involved with said homecoming queen's boyfriend, the captain of the football team. The story had heart. It had cattiness. And it had a heroine the likes of which had never previously been featured in one of MTV's scripted dramas.

Getting *Sweetheart's Dance* into production was a battle. Virtually everyone bristled at the idea of casting an overweight actress for the role of Bonnie. In fact, I remember having a conversation with the casting associate, who told me she wasn't sure they'd be able to find someone for the role, as if there weren't any talented actresses who happened to be overweight. Still, I fought to keep the story on the show. And luckily some other producers fought for the story—and the overweight lead actress—as well.

The *Undressed* storyline of *Sweetheart's Dance* (aka *Spring Fling* online) did get produced and was aired, with talented actress Jennifer Garms playing the lead role of Bonnie. The amount of mail I received regarding getting an overweight actress on an MTV show was incredible. I was taken aback by the number of letters from viewers who thanked me for creating a character who they could relate to. I was overwhelmed, not with pride, but with gratitude.

I realized that everything I'd suffered through in my past wasn't actually suffering at all. Sure, I'd hit some mighty big lows back in the day, and I'd done a lot of struggling. But I was realizing that everything I'd been through—everything I'd *lived* through—was now not only informing my writing, which had the potential to change and uplift lives, but also made me who I was in that moment.

It all made me . . . *me*.

Was it possible that up until now I'd been a spoiled brat? That by carrying around the angst of my childhood, the defensive reasoning for the excess weight and the endless excuses for just about everything else that went wrong in my life, I was holding myself back? That I was holding myself in the role of victim?

Not my mom.

Not the excess weight.

Not the loose skin, scars, or stretch marks.

But me. Gregg McBride. (Or *Greg* McBride according to the opening credits of *Epicenter*.)

Wow. That was a breakthrough. But one I wanted to be careful with, given my latest blast of clarity. After all, if I started blaming myself for past decisions, that wouldn't do anything to help my self-esteem. So instead of blame, I looked at everything in terms of ownership. And no, that doesn't mean my sister Lori and I deserved any of the machinations my mother and father put us through. But that was then. This is now.

BIG GIRLS DON'T CRY

It was through my writing that I'd discovered not only the power to heal myself, but the power to help others. I immediately took this newfound motivation and sat down to write my next feature-length screenplay. I titled it *Big Girls Don't Cry*. As you might guess, it has to do with three overweight high school girls who conspire to kidnap their school's prom queen wannabe in order to teach the students at their school a lesson in popularity they'll never forget.

Before too long, I got a call from an executive who worked for Saturday Night Live Films' shingle at the time. She had arranged for us to meet with one of the studio vice presidents at Paramount (where SNL Films had their deal). Mallory, the SNL Films executive, totally got my writing voice, loved the script, and was hoping she could set the project up at the studio. After the studio VP read the script, her office called to set up a meeting with Mallory and me.

This was it, I thought. My next big break. And the next way I might somehow touch people's lives for the better. Although *Big Girls Don't Cry* is an outlandish comedy, I made sure it also had a lot of heart and that, in the end, we like every character—even some of the high school bitchy types we love to hate through much of the script.

Showing up to the meeting, Mallory and I were both shaking with excitement. We entered the VP's office and sat down, ready to make a deal. Only this VP, who happened to be a "big girl" herself, took one look at me—a "thin male"—and immediately started listing off the reasons why she *hated* the script, most of them having to do with a thin guy having no business writing about large women. I think because of her own repressed prejudice about being overweight, she was projecting it all onto me, as if I'd written a script about larger girls as one big "look at the funny fat person" goof. Having been through what I've been through, nothing could have been further from the truth.

Mallory and I took turns trying to politely interrupt the VP to let her know about my personal backstory. I'd even thought to bring along a couple of "before" pictures to show her I knew what I was writing about. But she wouldn't let up, and basically tore our heads off, verbally.

I remember toward the end of the meeting thinking to myself, "Don't cry, Gregg. Just smile and nod. Like a Bobblehead." So that's what I did.

Smiled.

Nodded.

Bobblehead-ed.

Mallory's company was limited to making movies only under the Paramount banner, so there wasn't any other studio she could take the script to. This left me wondering if I ever should have written a feature script with three heavier girls as the lead characters.

As fate would have it, I soon got another call about the script from a different VP, this one worked for a company that had its deal at Sony Pictures. I wasn't looking forward to the meeting, worried it was going to be another disaster.

No matter. I would go. And I would let them know that I was still a big girl—I mean, um, *guy*—at heart despite what that morose Paramount VP said.

I knew I was screwed the minute I set foot in the Escape Artists' offices. Not only did the person I was meeting with have the title of "Vice *Princess*" (as opposed to Vice President), her assistant, a lovely girl named Jessica, happened to be overweight.

Oh, my gosh, I thought to myself. I'm screwed.

When I met Chrissy Blumenthal, the "Vice Princess" in question, I knew I was doubly screwed. She was blond, beautiful, and the epitome of a character in the script named Becka (a blonde cheerleader/prom queen wannabe whom everyone who reads the script initially loves to hate). I was sure I'd not only pissed off the assistant with the script, but Chrissy as well.

Despite the Hello Kitty paraphernalia strewn about her office, Chrissy took a terse tone with me from the get-go.

"I hesitated to call you in about your script," she told me. "I decided to have my assistant read it first to find out if she was offended or not."

I prepped my "Don't cry, Gregg" face as she took a long pause. And then?

"My assistant loved it," said Chrissy with a warm smile. "And so did I."

I was relieved, thrilled, elated—all in one. Chrissy not only understood my writing voice, but she got my intended message. And I'm happy to say she is a proponent of my writing and a good friend of mine to this day.

Sadly, a few options and near misses notwithstanding, the script *Big Girls Don't Cry* remains unproduced as of today. Hollywood is still too chicken to make a movie with "three fat girls" as the leads; also claiming they'd never find the right actresses for the roles.

Luckily for me, actresses like Melissa McCarthy (CBS's *Mike and Molly*) and Rebel Wilson (*Bridesmaids* and *Pitch Perfect*) are teaching Hollywood a thing or two about size prejudice. I still have hopes that *Big Girls Don't Cry* will eventually get produced. At this point I usually make a joke out of it—saying that I'm saving the project so I can direct it myself. Who knows? That just might happen.

WORTH THE WEIGHT

I continued to learn that being overweight was nothing to suppress. Not the before. Not the during. Not the after. And that being me, the real me (scars, stretch marks, and all), not only fueled my writing, but fueled my soul.

I was now free, really free, of the need to follow my mother's lead and try to be who I thought other people wanted me to be. With that came not only an enormous sigh of relief, but also an awakening of my spirit I had never known previously.

I'm not sure if putting on airs, if wanting the perfect swimsuit-ready body, or pretending to be someone I wasn't after moving to LA was a defense mechanism or simply a yearning to be loved and accepted. I make no qualms about still seeing life as a fat kid standing in a high school cafeteria, searching for where I can sit or where I'll fit in. Many people living on the West Coast would argue that being in Hollywood is like being in the world's biggest high school cafeteria. Still, I know a lot of that angst is in my head and, whether real or imagined, I'm no longer using that angst as an excuse not to be me.

These days if someone notices a scar, usually on my upper arms or legs, and asks about it, I tell them the reason it's there. I move my finger along the scar proudly, showing it off as if I were one of *The Price Is Right* models displaying a prize. That's what these scars are. *Prizes.*

At last, I'd reached a place where I wasn't wishing that things had been different in my past. I wasn't wishing I had been thin my entire life.

I wasn't wishing that my sister Lori and I were raised by different parents.

I wasn't wishing that I'd made quicker decisions in regard to dieting and nutrition.

All of that would have been a waste of time.

Along with this acceptance and embracing all of me—the "before" and "after"—came a healthy dose of self-forgiveness as well. Connecting with old friends from high school via Facebook reminded me of my exploits and attempts to fit in at all costs. Although I was still good friends with my girlfriend from high school, Amy, I was reminded of how I hurt her when I would choose to hang out with kids I deemed more popular than her. I was such a doofus.

Of course now I realize that my many charades in high school and beyond were defense mechanisms. I felt like no one would "accept" a fat kid as cool, so I surrounded myself with people who I thought were so cool that it would rub off on me a little. And I guess it did. But at whose expense?

There were other charades, including how I defended my mom and her reputation for being a slut, how I wrote notes supposedly from her to teachers and other authority figures whenever my sister and I needed that sort of thing, and then doing my best to maintain the illusion of family because our parents weren't around for weeks at a time.

I could stay bitter about all that now, or I could accept it and my behavior as that of a survivalist. That's what my therapist in San Francisco helped me realize—that what I was doing while being subjected to my parents' abuse was surviving. I tried to do the best for me and my sister. The best that I knew how to do in order to cope. That included lying. That included overeating. That included some mean and awful behavior toward Amy and others.

Today, instead of wincing, I just laugh about it and find the humor in every situation. For example, one time during high school my mother actually wrote a note to a high school teacher and I ended up being accused of forging that particular note. In other words, the school didn't recognize my mom's real signature as her authentic signature. Funny, right? I mean, why not laugh about it, rather than break down? Or break into a bag of Oreo cookies?

Do I have regrets? Sure. But do I know I was doing the best I knew how to do at the time? Absolutely. It's not like someone handed me a handbook titled *All the Right Decisions* and I never read it.

I've come to realize that before this time, when I would belabor, panic, or fill myself with regret over past decisions, I was acting like someone who owned a time machine that was out of service. No matter how filled with regret, no matter how remorseful, no matter how more *knowing* I am in this moment, there is no changing the past. Just like there's no changing the fact that I was morbidly obese for years and years and years.

Those are facts now. Plain and simple.

All of my "decisions" and actions from the past along with the circumstances I couldn't control make me who I am today. I've racked up a lot of life lessons. With the knowledge from those lessons, I'd likely make lots of decisions very differently today than I did back then.

The past does not make up who I am today, in this moment. But it does inform who I am today. Those past decisions and choices are a large part of what gives me my savvy, my humor, and my lust for life. And even, on occasion, some smarts.

And isn't that what life is all about? Living? Learning? Growing? For all that to happen, there has to be accepting. That's the real gift I've learned to give myself on a daily basis. Acceptance.

With this newfound clarity about loving and accepting all aspects of me came some newfound realities, and not all of them were pleasant. In all the mixed media messages we receive about dieting, it's always categorized as either "before" or "after." But as someone who has taken off more than 250 pounds (and re-lost another 100 pounds after re-gaining it initially), and who has now kept off those pounds for over a decade, I've come to learn that while there is some "before" and some "after," it's mostly the "during" that we "dieters" have to deal with.

Although we may reach our individual healthy goal weights, we may never *really* get to the point where we stop thinking about what food we put in our mouths and what kind of exercise we do for our bodies. It will all have to be adapted and changed as our bodies age, our metabolisms change, and we eventually begin to burn calories less efficiently.

These facts were, at first, a little disheartening. But then I looked around here in Hollywood. My beautiful former-supermodel-now-super-trainer friend, Ulli, thinks about what she consumes. Same goes for my "Vice Princess" friend Chrissy, who is now a writer in her own right. Does that mean these two, and others, don't enjoy their favorite food and drink? No. It just means they cut back when they need to, splurge moderately, and stay in great shape, mentally and physically.

Too many of us have bought the lie the media has been selling us over the years. We look at super thin and often super hot celebrities with lots of jealousy, thinking that they're blessed with perfect metabolisms and look amazing no matter how much they eat or how little exercise they do.

Looking good and, more importantly, feeling good take work. Plain and simple. That means I do have to think about what I eat every day, especially if I'm going to have a treat of some kind. It's all about balance. And the more I paid attention to how I felt and how my pants felt when fastening the waist, the more in touch I became with what the right choices are for me personally.

It's these same choices I make for my eating plan to this day.

A Typical Day on Gregg's Current Eating Plan

FIRST THING IN THE MORNING

1 large glass of Filtered Water (with 1 tbsp. Organic Lemon Juice)

BREAKFAST (POST-WORKOUT)

1 cup Kashi GoLean Crunch Cereal

1 medium Banana, sliced

1 cup 2% Lowfat Milk

1 Black Coffee

MID-MORNING

1 Black Coffee

LUNCH

Gregg's Best Lunch Salad Ever

(Recipe shared on page 267)

Sparkling Mineral Water

DINNER

Gregg's Beer'd Chicken

(Recipe shared on page 268)

Steamed Green Beans

(Sprinkled with Pepper, Granulated Garlic, and Balsamic Vinegar)

1/2 cup of Grape Tomatoes, sliced

Sparkling Mineral Water

AND THROUGHOUT THE DAY

Lots and lots of Filtered Water (room temperature)

What I've shared is a typical day, but I leave room for the occasional morning when I'll treat myself to a Chocolate Chunk Scone for breakfast, business lunches at restaurants, and even special occasion dinners. It's all about moderation as opposed to restriction. In other words, no more "last suppers."

One thing I am rather compulsive about is working out. I have found that after a lifetime of being on and off diets, my metabolism isn't the most efficient. And why should it be? I've virtually wrecked it with years and years of extreme dieting. I have found exercise to be the great balancer of all things, whether I've had a splurge meal the night before or stayed the course on my "normal" eating plan. I am committed to being at the gym every morning by 5:00. It doesn't matter if I was at a film premiere the night before or just catching up on watching TV shows on my DVR.

Gym.

Me.

Happening every morning. Even on holidays if my local gym is open.

The one time I will give my body time off from working out is if I'm traveling, but that is the only exception. And, for the record, I'm not encouraging anyone to emulate me—most experts will tell you that you need a day or two off from working out for your body's overall health. But for me, working out daily keeps me on track. So of all the compulsions I could have, I figure the persistent working out (and daily dose of two black coffees) is okay. For now. If and when I need to adapt this regimen, I will.

And yes, I have had to cut down on my splurges as my metabolism gets older. But that's a small price to pay for feeling good in my jeans. Or suit. Or sweats. Or pajamas.

In fact, I now use my clothes to monitor my weight rather than the scale. It's been years since I weighed myself. Even if I'm at the doctor's office for a physical, I tell the nurse who's weighing me that I do not want to know my weight. I've come to realize over the years that the scale is not my friend. If I'm up above my ideal weight, I get depressed and cheat. If I'm down below my ideal weight, I get happy and cheat.

230   WEIGHTLESS

Cycle.

Of.

Abuse.

So for me, my jeans let me know if I'm on target, weight-wise, or not. If they're a little snug, it's time to amp up the exercise and amp down the occasional splurge. If they're "just right," I know I'm staying the course with eating healthfully.

No, this way of living and eating and exercising isn't necessarily easy. It is something I always have to think about. But I've decided that I want to think about it and that I continually want to keep it in mind. Because one thing is undeniably true: No matter if you're getting dressed for the gym, for work, for a special occasion, or even for just watching TV and cuddling with your dog, any situation is made better when your clothes aren't cutting off your oxygen supply.

And isn't feeling as good as we look, no matter what the scale says, what it's all about? Abso-friggin'-lutely.

All that being said, I still had one major hurdle ahead of me. I knew if I didn't man up and address it, all of those other accomplishments would be for naught.

ANOTHER PERSPECTIVE
ON GREGG AT THIS TIME

By Chrissy Blumenthal, Gregg's Screenwriting Associate

At the height of my career as a development executive I was reading anywhere from two to four scripts a day, and even more on the weekends. Of all the scripts that crossed my desk, 99 percent were yawn inducing. They were either well-written but the story was nothing new, or the story was amazing but the writer was, well . . . let's just say challenged. Mainly the scripts were both: Horribly written with lackluster stories.

Needless to say, it was difficult to find a script that was both well-written and told a unique, entertaining story. So, when Gregg's script arrived, there was a good chance I wouldn't like it. The odds were stacked against him even before I turned to the first page. However, once I did, I couldn't stop turning the pages. *Big Girls Don't Cry* was funny, poignant, compelling, and beautifully written. I loved it! I couldn't wait to have Jessica, my assistant, set up a meeting.

The next morning I rushed into the office with my coffee and scripts in hand and just when I was about to ask Jessica to set up the meeting, I realized she very well could have been one of the characters in the script. I realized that maybe not everyone would find the script compelling, especially not people who were larger than the average size. To some people, fat might not always equal funny.

So instead of asking Jessica to set up the meeting, I had her read the script. I told her I needed to know if she found it offensive and assured her I wanted her honest opinion. A few hours later, she came into my office and told me she loved the script. "It's real," she said. So without any further delay, we set up a meeting with Gregg.

When Gregg walked into my office, I couldn't help but wonder how he found the voice to write *Big Girls Don't Cry*. He was neither *Big* nor was he a *Girl*. He was a good looking, slender young man. I was fascinated and couldn't wait to get inside his head. It didn't take long to find out how Gregg had found his voice. He was funny, charming, and eloquent. It was about halfway into our meeting that I learned he once weighed over 450 pounds. I was floored. Gregg blew me away not just with his wit and talent, but also with his strength, courage, and determination.

I promised him I would do whatever I could to get his script into the right hands, but while my Hollywood contacts fell in love with the script, the powers that be felt the project was too much of a risk. I respect the studio's decision of not wanting to offend overweight people—but perhaps they would have been revered instead for producing a story that was inspiring, compelling, raw, and real. To this day, *Big Girls Don't Cry* is one of my all-time favorite, unproduced screenplays.

Gregg and I may not have been able to make this film together, but we did form an unbelievable friendship. He will always be a great friend and a true inspiration in my life.

CHAPTER TWELVE

me, myself, and thigh(s)

Accepting myself was getting easier and easier. Accepting others was falling into place nicely as well. And with all that acceptance came enormous freedom.

Freedom from worry. Freedom from angst. Freedom from regret. And freedom from excess, which for me had always been defined by overeating.

At this point my father and I had a healthy enough "arm's-length" relationship. Ever the narcissist, it was still all about him, as illustrated by his Christmas newsletters, which always mentioned his third wife, her children he adopted, and my half-sister Nicole, but never anything about my sister Lori or me. But I was okay with that. I knew in my heart that Dad was, and always had been, doing the best he knew how to do—just like me. Just like all of us.

I even had occasional and positive email contact with Bonnie, my dad's second wife, now divorced and married to her second husband.

I was also keeping in touch with my sister, Lori, who is happily married and raising two beautiful daughters. I suppose being an amazing mom is Lori's way of un-doing some of the mental torture she suffered as a result of being raised by our particular parents. And I applaud her for that. The joy and brightness in her daughters' faces are proof that they're living very different childhoods from the one Lori and I had.

Still, Lori did not seem to want to discuss the past. She'd indulge me if I brought it up; in fact, she often had a better memory of a lot of the specific abuse that went on. But unlike me, she didn't seem to be at the same place of "acceptance" that I had gotten to. It was as if some part of her still had hope of being able to change or eliminate some of what we both survived.

I, on the other hand, was not only in touch with acceptance, but also in touch with my mom. Not a lot. Just a Christmas card here, or a recipe exchange there. Our contact was limited to about twice a year. And that contact was very comforting when I learned of her death one April.

My Uncle Garrett, my mother's brother, was the one who called to give us the news. No one else had thought to call me or Lori, not even my dad, who had apparently been told by my mom's other relatives. I wasn't completely shocked. From my mom's and my limited contact, I knew that she'd had kidney problems and had in fact been on dialysis in the recent years before her passing.

My last bit of contact with her had taken place the previous December. During a brief phone call she even mentioned that she might be coming out to the West Coast for a recipe contest she had entered. We hadn't made any firm plans to see one another, but we were both open to it. This gave me even more comfort upon learning of her death.

Knowing how much my mom's second husband Joe loved her— he really seemed to care about her very deeply—I decided to give him a call to pay my respects. I was doing so with an earnest heart, but I have to admit dialing him up was a stressful moment. Then, he answered.

"Hello?" said Joe, in his usual terse, drill sergeant-esque tone.

"Hi, Joe. It's me. Gregg."

No response.

"Gregg McBride?" I said, as if to jog his memory.

"I know who it is," he said gruffly.

"I just wanted to call and express my condolences on my mom's passing. I know how much you loved her."

"Yeah?" responded Joe even more tersely, "Well, I don't need to hear that from an ungrateful brat like you."

Click. Deafening silence indicated that Joe had hung up.

I'm grateful I was centered enough not to take Joe's words to heart. I reasoned that he was operating on a much different knowledge base about my mom's and my relationship that was far from factual. But to Joe, what my mother had shared with him was real.

So I did what anyone in LA would do. I went to the gym and worked out. No food binge was required to feel okay about this—a major achievement for this former 450-plus pound man.

Neither my sister nor I were invited to my mom's funeral. We weren't given any details about the funeral, the reading of the will, or anything else to do with those events before or after they took place. Lori and I both wondered what was going on. But given that Lori had had almost no contact with my mom and I'd had very little, it was fairly easy for us both to "move on," mentally.

DEARLY DEPARTED

About a year later, when my Uncle Garrett came to Los Angeles to visit his girlfriend's son, we met for dinner. I told him about my conversation with Joe. Garrett told me that after reading the obituary, which Joe had been in charge of getting written up by the local newspaper, they all (he and my mom's other remaining relatives) wondered what Joe knew and didn't know, and even whether, perhaps, Joe had "Gone a little off the deep end."

Now, honestly, my uncle was being pretty ignorant. My mother's side of the family had always ignored me and Lori. They do a more consistent job of staying in touch with my dad, post-divorce, than they do with my sister and me.

With me and Lori it always seemed to be a "don't ask, don't tell" policy. For example, why didn't my uncle spend a little less time wondering about Joe and instead question why Lori and I weren't present at the funeral?

The awkward dinner with Garrett and his questioning of Joe's mental state set me in motion. After a little online investigation, I was able to track down my mother's obituary. And boy, oh, boy was it an interesting piece of fiction.

DIANA S. GILBERT

OBITUARY

Diana S. Gilbert, 60, of Medford passed away on Tuesday April 27 at Virtua Memorial Hospital, Mt. Holly, NJ.

Born in Orlando, FL Diana resided in Carlisle, PA before moving to Medford seven years ago. Diana was an exciting and caring person who struck a positive note with everyone she met. She was incredibly intelligent, receiving her undergraduate degree from Radcliff and her MBA from Harvard. She proudly served her country for many years working with the State Department Air Force Intelligence and as a Department of Army Civilian employee. She was a seasoned traveler, spoke seven languages, and lived all over the world. She adopted and raised two orphans on her own—one from Germany and one from Iran. She was a gifted artist and a fascinating person who loved travel, good food, and the sea. She will be mourned and missed by her many friends locally and around the world.

Daughter of the late Albert and Theresa Clark; Diana is survived by her husband Joseph; one brother Garrett Clark; her adopted children Lori and Gregg.

Relatives and friends may call on Monday, May 3 from 9–10 a.m. at the Mathis Funeral Home. Funeral services will follow at 10:00 a.m.

Cremation will be held privately and at the convenience of the family.

I couldn't believe what I was reading.

I had to review the obituary several times before it sank in, especially the part about not only *me* being adopted (from Iran?!), but my sister Lori being adopted from Germany.

Whoa.

Just for kicks, let's go over this obituary again. But now, I'm going to point out a few of the inaccuracies.

DIANA S. GILBERT

OBITUARY

Diana S. Gilbert, 60 *(my mom's lie age of the minute)*, of Medford passed away on Tuesday April 27 at Virtua Memorial Hospital, Mt. Holly, NJ.

Born in Orlando, FL, Diana resided in Carlisle, PA before moving to Medford seven years ago. Diana was an exciting and caring person who struck a positive note with everyone she met. She was incredibly intelligent, receiving her undergraduate degree from Radcliff *(my mother never went to college)* and her MBA from Harvard *(this was my dad's degree, not my mom's)*. She proudly served her country for many years working with the State Department Air Force Intelligence *(my mom a spy? Hardly! She was a glorified secretary and never one for the State Department Air Force Intelligence)* and as a Department of Army Civilian employee. She was a seasoned traveler, spoke seven languages *(my mom has always told this lie, yet never spoke any languages except English)* and lived all over the world. She adopted and raised two orphans on her own *(Wowza!)*—one from Germany and one from Iran *(Really?!)*. She was a gifted artist and a fascinating person who loved travel, good food, and the sea. She will be mourned and missed by her many friends locally and around the world.

Daughter of the late Albert and Theresa Clark; Diana is survived by her husband Joseph; one brother Garrett Clark; her adopted children Lori and Gregg *(that's us—only we're not adopted)*.

Relatives and friends may call on Monday, May 3 from 9–10 a.m. at the Mathis Funeral Home. Funeral services will follow at 10:00 a.m.

Cremation will be held privately and at the convenience of the family.

After sharing the obituary with Lori, she and I both realized we would never escape the legacy of our mother's lies. It hurt us both to read that obituary, perhaps because we had both thought our mom would "come clean" on her death bed. But why would we expect that after a lifetime of denying our existence (our *real* existence), she would finally break down and tell the truth?

I think even more mind-boggling to my sister and me was that people like our Uncle Garrett and even our dad had become complacent with our mother's lies. Would no one question that obituary, not even my uncle who did travel to and attend my mom's funeral? Would no one come to our defense or wonder why we weren't included?

Those crimes of ignorance extend much further back than our mom's funeral. Our dad knew what my mom was up to while we were young. My mom's relatives had to have had a clue as well. And yet no one—*no one*—intervened on behalf of the children. No one came to our defense. No one even came or called to check if we were surviving.

But survive we did. In my case, through *thick* and now through *thin*.

My sister still shudders whenever the subject of the obituary comes up. And I have to admit, it's unsettling to me to read it to this day. But back when I first found it, after the initial shock wore off, I decided that her obituary wasn't going to set me back.

I said to Lori that in a strange way, the obituary gave us proof not only of our mother's deceit, but also of her sickness. Lori and I have both had a hard time convincing those closest to us that our mother was capable of such heinous lies. Now we had proof. The obituary.

The most hilarious part was the claim that I was adopted from Iran. At least I assume I'm the Iranian one since the sequence of Lori's and my names falls in line with her being adopted from Germany and me from Iran, according to the obituary.

The obituary reminded me of the times in my life when I actually questioned whether or not I was really adopted, and when I even asked my dad about it in an effort to know the truth. Of course, the funny thing is, I'm the spitting image of both my mom and my dad. Eyes. Nose. Bone structure. This apple did not fall far from the tree. But I refused to let that gene pool control me any further than that.

I knew that with a printout of the obituary, I was holding the final piece of the puzzle. The puzzle of me being a whole person.

I decided at that moment that I wasn't going to give my mother, or what she'd done over the years, any more power over my psyche, my eating, the way I interacted with others, or my life in general. I was reclaiming my power, or, perhaps, claiming it for the first time. I knew that meant finding a way of not only accepting my mother and all of her actions, but also to love her. I was determined to find a way to think of my mother with love. For my own good. Not for Joe's. Not for my dad's. Not for my uncle's. And not even for my sister Lori's well being. But for my own.

This is when I turned to my memory banks. I scanned my internal databases and scoured my recollections for a pleasant one involving my mother. To my surprise, I eventually found it. And it made me smile.

GREGG'S HAPPY MOTHER MEMORY

While attending Lynn University, I had discovered my favorite new alcoholic beverage. You may not be surprised to learn that it wasn't beer that caught my taste buds' fancy. Nope. For this plus-sized young man, it was Piña Coladas. Frozen, creamy deliciousness. A lot like ice cream, but with a kick. And for me it was less about the buzz from the rum than it was a love affair with the whipped cream slathered on top.

Well, for some reason I felt compelled to let my mom know that I had discovered "my favorite new drink" when writing home.

That following summer, when I flew back to Germany between semesters, my mother picked me up at the airport. I was in a grumpy mood at the time. I didn't want to leave the new friends I'd met at Lynn for a whole summer. I was also wearing a cast after a misstep that resulted in me stumbling down a flight of stairs and breaking my foot.

Anyway, upon getting in my mom's car in the airport parking lot, she reached behind the passenger seat and produced a cold thermos. Inside the thermos were freshly made Piña Coladas, whipped up by my mom just before coming to the Frankfurt International Airport to pick me up.

She didn't want any for herself. It was all for me. I remember drinking the Piña Colada from the thermos's cup and laughing with my mom as I regaled her with the story of how my foot cast came to be. It was a brief moment of mother-son bonding. But a moment nonetheless.

A moment that still brings, and will always bring, a smile to my face.

To this day, whenever I think of my mom I don't immediately recall the years and years of abuse. Nor do I recall her claiming that I'm adopted or that I have a disease that makes me fat. I don't remember her reputation as the town tramp, and I don't remember her being appalled when I asked her what my first words were as a kid.

Instead, I remember my mom handing me that thermos full of Piña Colada. And for me, that's enough.

This doesn't mean I've suppressed my history with my mother or what my sister and I endured. I never want to forget that. It not only helps to define me, but it helps me be a more compassionate person. Those memories don't keep me from being who I am today. They actually enhance who I am. For I am not a victim. I am a *Gregg*. And I choose to think of Piña Coladas when I think of my mother. With or without whipped cream.

Finding my mother's obituary online was definitely the crescendo in what's been a lifelong journey to lasting health, both physical and mental. What I read in that obituary could have triggered all sorts of things, including a slow progression back up the scale to over 450 pounds.

Instead, that obituary tested my resolve, as well as my compassion. I think that for the most part, my mom really did believe her own lies. I'm sad she lived a life in which she thought she couldn't be herself and, instead, had to lie and deceive people, including her second husband, to feel accepted. If my mom were here now, I'd give her a big hug. And then, perhaps, I'd treat her to a Piña Colada.

I realized that at last I was free. And not because my mom was gone, but because I knew who I was and didn't need her, or her obituary, to validate my existence in this life.

I'm not sure if I believe in heaven or hell. My belief in any kind of afterlife remains just as undefined. But about six months after my mother passed away, I happened to meet someone who I eventually recognized to be the love of my life. The best way I can describe this person's love for me is to compare it to the way that Joe loved my mother.

I'd never met someone who was more devoted, more accepting, and dedicated to someone than Joe was toward my mom. It makes me sad that my mom didn't realize that even without all of her lies, Joe would have still loved her just as much, not in spite of her flaws, but because of them.

I'm happy and relieved to report that this is the kind of love I have in my marriage. And deep within my heart, I'd like to think my dearly departed mom might have had something to do with our meeting. Even if not, the fact that the thought brings a little more warmth to my heart when I think about my mom is a good thing. After all, I don't want my only pleasant thoughts of my mother to have to do with Piña Coladas!

With this freedom and ease I allowed myself in regard to my mom and our shared history, I realized that I'd finally let go of my remaining excess weight, the excess weight I needed to release (or "lose") most of all. Not the physical weight, but the *mental* weight. I am not just 250 pounds thinner, but I'm now also much lighter in the head.

This clarity, release, and acceptance were not typical conclusions for someone who always blamed himself for not doing certain things (losing weight, dropping pretenses, etc.) sooner in life, as if I was on a crazy game show on which I needed to beat some imaginary clock. But, had I not lived through every moment of my life up to now, in exactly the way that I did, I don't think I would have drawn these kinds of conclusions or achieved this kind of relief.

For the first time in a long time—perhaps *ever*—I realized that, at long last, I was . . . *weightless.*

ANOTHER PERSPECTIVE
ON GREGG AT THIS TIME

By Kim Pedersen, Gregg's Longtime Friend

I met Gregg in Tallahassee when he was attending Florida State University and had developed a couple of student films that were shown at a local theater. Our mutual friend, Don, who was moving away from Tallahassee, introduced us, thinking it would be nice for Gregg and me to become friends in Don's absence.

I don't remember the exact time or place we met. What I do remember most about meeting Gregg was his sense of humor and his creative nature. He also happened to be a very large person. For the record, I was a shy 5'3" blonde girl living with her parents who never had to diet or ever had a weight problem. Gregg and I did hit it off and soon we were regularly going to the movies and out to eat together.

My mother would always have dinner prepared well in advance, so when Gregg would call and ask me to go get something to eat at the last minute, it would be somewhat frustrating for my mother as she had planned on having me at dinner already. It wasn't so much that I wouldn't be at dinner, but her concern over preparing too much food. Because this happened so often, it quickly became an inside joke. Gregg even made a movie poster for me as a gift titled, "Supper Interrupter"—a scary movie with the villain asking the girl to dinner after too much food is taken out of the freezer. *Horrors!* I still have the framed poster in my home. While it has faded over the years, it still makes me laugh.

One time my parents went to dinner at a local French restaurant that Gregg and I had gone to just days earlier. One of the servers there, who I happened to know, asked my father who I had been dining with. I believe my father was very aware that this server's "curiosity" was piqued by Gregg's size. My dad was a man of 6'2" and weighed over 300 pounds himself. He just said, "Oh, that was Gregg. He's a movie producer." That took my nosy friend by surprise and ended the conversation. My father had a great sense of humor and would often use it to deal with his own weight issues.

Some years later I remember visiting Gregg in New York and he proudly showed me where he lived and worked. We went to dinner at a fashionable little restaurant on the West Side. When we walked into the restaurant we were met with some interesting stares. I imagine they were surprised to see someone of Gregg's size paired up with someone of mine. At some point during the meal I got it into my head that I should pique their curiosity by giving them something more to think about besides our contrasting sizes. So with my back to this particular table of onlookers, as well as most of the restaurant, I started with what could be described as an enthusiastic rambling monologue of how Gregg should cast his next movie. It went something like, "You should go with an unknown actress, not a Meg Ryan or a Julia Roberts." This went on for several minutes. Gregg could see their faces but I could not. Now they were straining their necks to try and hear what I was saying and their wheels were turning while trying to figure out who this movie mogul was. That was great fun.

Gregg eventually moved out West to San Francisco and I went to visit him there for a few days as well. This was after Gregg had had the surgery to remove the excess skin after his weight loss. I don't recall if he showed me his scars. But I do remember that he had to remind himself to stand up straight as the surgery had tightened the skin on his stomach. So to prevent himself from slouching and ending up with poor posture he had to force himself to stand tall.

As always we had a lot of laughs. During my visit we went out with some of his friends, walked along the Marina Green, went to an art festival, and spent a fun-filled day in Sausalito. By the end of the trip we had a list of the top ten funny things that happened during the visit and I wish I remembered what they were now.

I do remember it was the first time I ever had sushi. Gregg took me to a place where we sat at a counter and sushi came by on a conveyer belt and you took the plate of sushi that appealed to you off the belt as it passed by. I had never seen or eaten anything like it. What a blast. It was all about the sushi, and it was probably the first time Gregg and I dined together that our appearances were not part of the meal.

Those are all old memories from years ago and we have both moved on. I am still a 5'3" small blonde chick, but I am not shy anymore. Gregg still has a killer sense of humor and a smile to match. His creativity has helped him evolve into the person he's become. He truly is a self-made man. I never knew the details of the hardships he endured in his youth before now, though I suspected his weight was baggage he carried with him as a result of a difficult time in his childhood. But who was I to pry? And besides, how do you ask somebody, "Why are you the way you are?" None of my business, right? If he wanted to talk about it, he would have told me.

Well, now, with this book, he has told everyone. I don't think I know anyone who has lost so much and gained so much in order to become such a warm and open person. I don't mean the weight. I mean that he has taken his life from a beginning that was not a loving and nurturing environment and left it behind to become a person who embraces life, looks at the good in life, expects good things, and has gained good things in his own life.

Gregg and I have come in and out of each other's lives several times over the years and today remain good friends who regularly talk on the phone, email, text, and Skype about the issues in our lives. As Gregg reminds me, there will always be some issues we are dealing with and are challenged by, but we work through them and we don't focus on them. We choose to see the joy that life brings and we strive to attract more of that joy into our own lives.

Maybe what we see in another person is what we choose to see in ourselves. Through the years I always saw Gregg's sense of humor and creativity shine through. We focused on the laughter. A sense of humor can definitely help a person get through tough times. I look forward to the next visit with Gregg, whenever and wherever that will be, and I am sure we will sit down to enjoy a meal and laugh and laugh and laugh.

EPILOGUE

the big reveal

In an instant all the flashbacks from the past are over. My childhood. The broken movie theater seat. The desperate attempts at losing weight. The equally desperate attempts at keeping it off. And the longing for acceptance—the acceptance that ended up being inside me all along.

No time to wonder about that now. My eyes are starting to adjust to the bright lights I've been instructed to walk toward.

As I strut forward, I hear the song I requested be played as I enter ("Ride," sung by country artist Martina McBride). Reconnecting with feeling weightless, I decide to be myself—which means letting my silliness flow.

I'm now not just strutting, but walking to the beat as if I were a model on some runway in Milan. Reaching an "X" on the floor in front of me, I stop and assume a model-esque pose. But I decide that's not enough, so I ask, "Am I not here for the modeling segment?"

I've done it. I've made my entrance. And here I am, after a lifetime of adventures up and down the scale, a guest of nutrition expert Joy Bauer, along with Kathie Lee Gifford and Hoda Kotb, on NBC's *Today* show for a "Joy's Fit Club" segment. These popular segments feature people who have lost 100 or more pounds by relying solely on diet and exercise.

It turns out when I was "shoved" into the dark office, Anne Curry's while she was still with the *Today* show, Joy Bauer had done so in order to hide me from the approaching hosts. She didn't want Kathie Lee or Hoda to see me before the on-air segment so that their shock at seeing me "thin" (after seeing my "before" pictures on the air) would be significant and genuine. And it was.

I was very nervous about my "national TV debut," but I knew it was my chance to be my authentic self and not someone like my mother who would have acted like a "pretend person," thinking it would make the audience more responsive. When I saw the "before" picture that was being featured, me without a shirt at over 450 pounds, I remarked candidly, "Wow, everyone has just seen my man boobs. I feel like I was nursing America."

Responding to me being so straightforward, Kathie Lee made a comment about the blond highlights in my hair, saying, "Now America can see your highlights."

Not missing a beat, I said, "You know what? I lost 250 pounds and went blond."

I like to think my authenticity helped the segment given that Kathie Lee, Hoda, and Joy were all giggles as I showed them my old sixty-inch waist belt and then proceeded to wrap all three of them up in it. When I told them I wanted to wrap them all in my belt, Kathie Lee responded, "Get in line, buddy!"

As the segment ended, Kathie Lee took the belt and readied it to pretend to spank me. So naturally I leaned over and let her do it. Quite a difference from the belt beatings I used to receive as a child. Needless to report, there were no tears.

I have to admit that appearing on the *Today* show was one of the happiest moments of my life. Not just because of the fun of appearing on TV and getting lots of phone calls, emails, and Facebook posts from friends who saw me, but because I knew that I was being me and owning every aspect of myself.

The elation about the *Today* show adventure extended far beyond the day it was televised. The amount of messages and posts I received from virtual strangers after my debut was incredible and so uplifting. I realized that by appearing on the show, I was not only representing a segment of society that wanted to be recognized for more than just their size, but also giving hope to anyone who thought they'd gone down too dark of a path to return from.

If I can do it, anyone can do it. And I mean *anyone*. I wanted anyone watching the show, and want anyone reading these words, to know that. I am only as strong and equally as vulnerable as you are. And this was proven by every message I received after appearing on the show. I got as much uplift from hearing from people as they claimed to have gotten from me. This made and continues to make my public unveiling such a gift, and a happily reciprocal one.

Along with Kathie Lee, Hoda, and everyone who works behind the scenes at the morning show, I must give props to one Ms. Joy Bauer, a person who truly walks her talk. Today, years since that and even a few other *Today* show appearances, I am happy to call Joy not just an inspiration, but also a friend. Her personality sparkles. And for a thin chick she really understands the dieter's psyche and offers paths for all of us to get healthier in the sanest ways possible.

Everything I lived through led up to the *Today* show appearance. Not only my triumphs, but also my failures, as well as the other things I lived through as a child that weren't caused by my own actions. My mom. My dad. My eating, past and present. All of those are aspects of who I am today and, I would like to think, have come together to make me an empathetic person with a personal mission to get the word out that real health—physical and mental—is possible for everyone.

I work to communicate this message through my blog, my Facebook page, and anytime someone brings up the topic of weight loss or healthy eating. Anyone who's met me knows that once I get started on the subject, it's hard to shut me up.

And that brings us to the part where I tell you that if I can face and overcome crazy odds, you can too. I'm not going to lie to you. I'm a work in progress. Even as I write this, I would like to stop typing, go to the kitchen, and eat a bag of cookies. But I choose not to.

And that's what life is, I think. A series of choices. Key word? *Series*. That means along with all the choices for us to make in this present moment, there are millions more ahead of us. So it's really not worth questioning the choices we've made in the past. I'm not saying we shouldn't acknowledge those choices, after all that's how we learn. But that stuff is all in the past. There's nothing we can do but look forward and see ourselves as the survivors and thrivers that we are.

This same message is summed up beautifully by my amazing friend Jaxon Blumenthal who, at just eleven years old, was diagnosed with a rare form of liver cancer. Jax not only had to face a series of brutal treatments and medical challenges, but eventually underwent a successful liver transplant.

Before, during, and after that grueling process, Jax's spirit remained bright. He and his sister Calli (children of my friends Jason and Chrissy Blumenthal—the same Chrissy featured in Chapter Eleven of this book) have always exhibited star quality. One of Jax's many talents includes songwriting and performing. And as it happens, Jax penned a song called "Weightless" not too long ago. These lyrics are dear to my heart (as is Jaxon). I'd like to share them with you, now that you've been on my life journey with me.

weightless

By Jaxon Blumenthal

You might try to bring me down but I will rise above it.
You try to push me to the ground but you should just forget it.

I've grown stronger and finally know my way,
Unlike yesterday.
Today I feel weightless. No fear inside of me.
I'm unstoppable now.

Today I feel weightless. Like I can just be free.
From here on I'm unbound.

I'm weightless.

Some days it might feel real hard but I just keep on pushing.
When it's raining pain and fear let it flow into the ocean.

I've grown braver and finally know my way,
Unlike yesterday.
Today I feel weightless. No fear inside of me.
I'm unstoppable now.

Today I feel weightless. Like I can just be free
From here on I'm unbound.

I'm weightless.

Today I feel weightless. I'm unstoppable now.

Like me and like Jaxon, you have everything it takes to survive, everything it takes to succeed, everything it takes to take off (regardless of how you define "take off").

No matter what your scale registers (yesterday, today, or tomorrow), you—and everyone else reading this—have the power to be *weightless*.

what's in it for you?

Am I a medical professional? No. Am I a trained therapist? No. Am I a nutrition or exercise expert? Not necessarily. But you can count me in as a health enthusiast and someone who has lived through the journey of being morbidly obese.

When people find out what I used to weigh they often ask for my advice—whether they want to lose five or 100-plus pounds. Because this is a topic of conversation with both strangers and people who are close to me, I decided to share my best advice here.

Whether you want to initiate changes for yourself, or whether you want to know more in order to help out a loved one, this is real-world advice I share from the bottom of my heart and both sides of the scale.

As I tell everyone who asks me for advice, use what resonates with you. Ignore what doesn't. Mine has been a unique, individual journey full of highs (450-plus pounds) and lows (eating out of the garbage can). One thing I can assure you of is that my journey was authentic. I lived it. And because of this, I felt compelled to share it.

Please be smart about what journey to a healthy weight you decide to take. Make decisions that are right for you, and include your doctor in the process. It makes no sense to look good on the outside if you're not equally as healthy on the inside.

That being said, here goes . . .

If I had bought a book like this years ago when I was still heavy, I would have flipped to this bonus section without reading the rest of the book. If that's what you've done, I'm all for it. Fact is, we never know in advance where the answers lie in regard to our individual paths to becoming weightless.

It could happen while watching an overweight, out-of-breath actor on *Saturday Night Live*. Or, perhaps, when a coworker glibly suggests that you "Just stop eating so much!" Whenever and however it happens for you, run with it. There is no one "diet cure" for all people. Our personal paths to gaining the excess weight happened for individual reasons. Perhaps it was a survival method. Perhaps it was a defense tactic. Or maybe it just happened because ice cream tastes so good.

But no matter. This is the moment when everything can change, when you can finally begin to shed the unwanted pounds and the no-longer-serving-you *mental* weight, and feel good doing it. It all starts with one simple question:

DO YOU WANT TO LOSE YOUR EXCESS WEIGHT?

If your answer is "Yes," then congratulations. You're going to do it. Yes, you read that right. You. Are. Going. To. Do. It. How do I know? Because you just told me that you want to.

If, by chance, you answered "No" to the question above, then so be it, and learn to live in as healthy a way as you can with your excess weight. And keep asking yourself the question. If the answer changes, turn back to this page and read on.

For the rest of you? Let's move forward, shall we?

I'm going to restate the good news: This is going to be the time that you do it. Why? Because you *want* to.

But first, some bad news. When it comes to taking off and keeping off the excess weight, there are no magic wands, tricks, or shortcuts. If someone or some organization tells you there are, turn around and head in another direction.

At the end of the day, taking off excess weight, no matter how much, is easy. Yes, you read that right—*easy*. In fact, it can be done in just four simple steps:

Gregg's Four Non-Tricks for Losing Weight

1. Eat less
2. Move more
3. Drink plenty of water
4. Get plenty of sleep

I'm going to pause to let you finish rolling your eyes.

Okay, so I know you've heard, read, or otherwise been pounded with most of these tenets for losing weight before. But I've found that while we can recite these methods, we don't actually embrace them, even though there's not that much to comprehend.

These are simple steps for losing excess weight because losing and keeping off weight is simple. We have to work at it. But the work's worth doing. And don't forget your answer to my earlier question. You *want* to take off the weight, right? Well, there's no time like the present. And this is all a really big *present* you're going to give to yourself.

In this bonus section, I'm going to share some ideas, recipes, and workout tips that have worked for me as well as people I know personally and people who have written to me with their success stories.

In addition to what I'm going to share here you can also visit JustStopEatingSoMuch.com anytime for motivation, inspiration, and even the occasional rant. I also post a lot of recipes, ideas, and inspirational quotes along with some of the latest healthy living news on the Just Stop Eating So Much Facebook page at facebook.com/juststopeatingsomuch. These are both free resources you can turn to anytime.

Now, let's go over the four "non-trick" ways to take off weight in more detail, shall we?

1. EAT LESS

The first step to achieving lasting health is the realization that there's not one sure-fire eating plan (or diet) that works for everyone. We all have different lifestyles that create different challenges. We also all have different tastes and some of us have food allergies we need to pay attention to.

When choosing a weight-loss plan, choose something that works for your life, your budget, and your family if you have one. You don't want to be fixing one kind of meal for yourself and an entirely different meal for your spouse and/or kids. Sure, you can add to their meals with some starches or even some healthier desserts, but for the most part, it's going to be easiest to stick with one menu and then adapt dishes slightly as needed.

Before deciding which eating plan might be right for you, I urge you to get to your doctor for a checkup, and let him or her know you're about to embark on a weight-loss plan. It's essential you get the medical care and advice necessary to make this a healthy journey. What good is losing weight if your teeth rot out, you get too skinny, you look gaunt or malnourished, or you have no energy? Getting rid of the excess weight should be as much about feeling good as it is about looking good.

For the record? You look good now. In this moment. I'm of the mindset that all of us are supermodels—male or female. And you are no different. Hating yourself or your looks is not a successful mindset to embark on this journey. Instead, love yourself in this minute, just as you are.

Why? Well consider who you'd rather help out with a favor—a friend you love, a total stranger, or even an enemy? As people with a dieter's mindset, we often see ourselves as the enemy. But we're not the enemy. We are incredible human beings even if our pants are a little tight or we can't fit into a Size 2 (which, for the record, is a size I'm not even sure my seven pound dog can fit into).

Stop with the negative mind chatter. And don't hit back with "It's hard to turn off the negative voices." Just turn them off. Period. Think of it as changing a channel. Just do it. And if you happen to accidentally switch back to the "beat yourself up network," then switch the channel again. Keep doing it until not mentally beating yourself up becomes the norm. Trust me, if I can stop beating myself up, anyone can.

As you can see, I assume a somewhat "tough love" approach to weight loss and positive change. That's because I believe in keeping things simple. Yes, you may have some issues in your past (like I did), or some issues with your love life (like I did), or some issues with your current interpersonal relationships (like I did), or some issues with your own self (like I did and still *do*), but so what? None of that has anything to do with the question at hand:

DO YOU WANT TO LOSE YOUR EXCESS WEIGHT?

And, yes. It really *is* that simple. If you want to feel better in your clothes, feel more confident in both work and social settings, not feel your heart racing or your breath quickening when you're just walking from one end of the room to the other, and to enjoy real food for the first time in your life, then *yes*—you want to lose your excess weight.

For me, the word and the concept of "dieting" has gotten me into trouble. This is mainly because for years and years I lived my life "on" a diet or "off" of one, and when I was "off" I would eat insanely as if I would never be able to have ice cream or cookies again.

Now depending on how much weight you want to take off, you may actually need a diet. But try and think of it more as an eating plan, one that can breathe and grow with you as necessary.

Try not to think to yourself, "I can never have [insert name of forbidden food here] again." Instead think, "I choose not to have this certain food today. But maybe I'll have it in a healthy portion on the weekend."

See what I did there? I gave you permission to have chips, ice cream, or whatever you want, *from time to time*. But right now? Let's find a plan that works for you, gives you the necessary nutrients, helps you keep to your food budget, and becomes a plan you can live with until you, too, are in the "average sizes clothes store," picking out your new pair of jeans.

Don't get me wrong. I'm not giving you permission to cheat. In fact, I'd like you to eliminate the word "cheat" from your vocabulary. Much like being "on" or "off" a diet, the word "cheating" sets those of us with a dieter's mentality up for trouble. Mainly because we equate cheating with excess. For example, "If I'm *cheating* with ice cream today, I better have as much as I can eat, since I won't be *cheating* with ice cream next week."

Cheating, bad. Eating, never bad. As long as it's in moderation.

And please, I beg of you, forget the notion of "cheat days." Oh, boy, can this concept lead us down a dark (and fat) path. People with a thin (healthy) mentality never cheat. When they want the cookie, they eat the cookie. But a lot of the time it's just one cookie. Or even a half of a cookie. Cheating is a concept that has kept us fat. Time to remove it from our vocabulary, and ban it from our way of doing things. Period.

When coming to grips with living in balance and eating in balance, I was reminded of my "research phase" back at Macy's in New York City, when I "secretly" stalked my coworker Charlene and vice president Alan in order to find out how thin people live their lives. Later, when I mentioned my "thin stalking" behavior during a phone call to Petra, my friend who lives in the Kansas City area, she didn't balk or make fun of me. Instead, she told me that she did the same thing once.

In fact, Petra revealed that she had not only observed thin people, but also turned the table and observed fat people, too. Petra shared her findings with me and I was literally floored. Her list is pure genius in regard to simple truths that those of us with a dieter's mentality might be out of touch with.

Don't believe me? Here are Petra's astute observations:

Observing Thin and Fat People

By Petra Allen

OBSERVING THE THIN PERSON

- Thin people *never* skip meals.
- Thin people know how much they can eat at a meal and fill their plates accordingly. If they're still hungry, they eat more. If they're full with one bite left on the plate, they don't eat it.
- Thin people don't think about food all the time. They simply pack or order a lunch and eat it without much thought.
- Thin people eat regularly, every day, and always at regular times. If their schedule is off and it's getting late for a meal, they get cranky.
- Thin people don't always eat dessert. Yet sometimes they do. They ask their bodies first, *is there still room?* They know they can have dessert tomorrow, if they have room.
- Thin people eat the birthday cake at the office, *one piece*, and then they are done. They don't think about it anymore. There will be another cake, another birthday.
- Thin people move. They are not sluggish. It helps that they get regular fuel from regular eating. They may or may not go to the gym, but they are *active*. And they enjoy it.

- Thin people breathe. They get outside. Thin people often have bright eyes. They have fat in their diets.
- Thin people have random treats in the house at random times, but don't need to eat them all at the same time to get rid of them. The treats could actually stay around for weeks!
- Thin people don't have "bad days" and "good days" or "on days" and "off days" when it comes to food.
- Thin people just eat, naturally, instinctively. They listen to their bodies without thinking, just like they go to bed when it's time and use the bathroom when it's time.
- Thin people do *not* weigh themselves daily or even weekly.
- Thin people enjoy their food; eating is an *enjoyable* thing.
- Thin people think of food as a friend.

OBSERVING THE FAT PERSON

- Fat people skip meals.
- Fat people *always* want to clean the plate. They will even trick themselves by using smaller plates.
- Fat people think about food ALL the time. *What can I eat? When can I eat it? Should I eat it?* Personally, when I'm having lunch, I'm planning dinner, and sometimes even planning the next day's breakfast.
- Fat people eat randomly, if their schedule allows. *Irregularly.* They'll try to *not* eat to save calories.
- Fat people think "to eat or not to eat" dessert is the ultimate question. The magnitude of this question for a fat person is hard to explain. It will actually keep him or her up at night.
- Fat people go through turmoil over whether they can or cannot have the birthday cake brought to the office. This turmoil will likely ruin their day, whether they decide to have the cake or not.
- Fat people like sitting. Exercise is something that *must* be done and when they do it, it is often overdone and frantic and very irregular.
- Fat people like the indoors, because they often don't have the energy to play outside, because they are *dieting*. Their eyes aren't

very bright. They hate their fat bodies and hate having to diet and
they are eating all "non-fat" yucky stuff!

- Fat people can't have any treats around the house. Their
roommates, significant others, or whole family must suffer. That's
it! No *ifs*, *ands*, or *buts* about it.

- Fat people judge all days as "good or bad" and "on or off,"
depending on what they did or didn't eat. Sometimes they confuse
this with feelings about themselves, good or bad.

- Fat people think of food as the enemy.

My beautiful friend Petra's brilliant observations not only make for a
handy guide to life, especially for this guy who used to be consumed by
being "on" or "off" a diet, but also offer helpful reminders about how I
want to think and not think about food. It's this kind of mentality that
my current eating plan reflects. Yours can reflect the same.

Many of us need to learn or re-learn portion control for the first
time. This is what an eating plan (or "diet") can help us do. So look at
your chosen eating plan, whether a public one like Weight Watchers
or a private one that your doctor gives you, as a tool—something that
provides guidelines and helps you re-learn how to eat healthily.

If it helps, you might want to adapt my "Hollywood approach"
to all this. As someone who works in the showbiz industry I see what
it takes for actors and models to look as good as they do. Sure, there
are some people who "can eat whatever they want," but 99.9 percent
of today's performers work out a lot and eat very healthily. And when
they have to look a certain way for a role, they're assigned a special
diet and workout regimen.

Our version of this doesn't necessarily come with a personal
chef or trainer. But we can think of our eating plans as our road
maps to getting ready for our role, in this case, our role in life. Think
I'm kidding? I'm not. This all really is a mindset. Much as I likened

myself to a racehorse with blinders on while initially taking off the 250-plus pounds, it also helps for me to think of myself as a celebrity who's on a special diet for a special role. And you know what? If mental tactics like that can help, then why not use them?

When choosing a diet, pick one that makes sense nutritionally, and one that gives you lots of choice. "Choice" being the keyword. Personally I'm no fan of diets that offer prepackaged foods, be they frozen or freeze dried. Besides all the additives, preservatives, and artificial ingredients these "meals" often contain, I believe these types of prepackaged foods can set us dieters up for trouble. The first meal during which we find ourselves needing to order "real" food, we have the potential to go nuts. By contrast, if we're on a diet like Weight Watchers, which offers every food choice you can imagine, we can pick and choose (and portion) to our heart's content.

I'm not endorsing Weight Watchers or any specific diet. I know what works for me. You need to find what works for you, which might even be a combination of dieting methods. You're a unique individual. Find something that works for *you*.

Don't get me started on liquid diets, juice fasts, meal replacement bars, and other mumbo-jumbo that we're fed as being the answer to the weight loss we've been looking for. Need a snack? Reach for an apple, which is just as convenient as one of those so-called "nutrition bars."

This is real life. We should eat real food.

This shouldn't be about "giving up everything until I reach my goal." Because guess what? As it is with me, it's likely you're always going to have to think about what you eat. We never really arrive at the "after" of dieting. Otherwise, we'd gain it all back.

Find a plan you can live with. And I mean *live* with. Today. Tomorrow. At your cousin Sheila's wedding. And when you're wearing stylish clothes that look and feel good, you're going to have heads turning.

The funny thing is that most of us have been on so many diets that we don't even need a prescribed diet to make the weight loss happen. We've pretty much learned what equates to a diet-friendly breakfast, lunch, and dinner. But many of us do like to have specific guidelines (or meal plans) in front of us, especially when starting out. So I'm all for it, as long as it's healthy.

Whichever plan you choose, along with getting your doctor's "okay," I also urge you to invest in a small food scale, measuring cups, and measuring spoons. This is something I'm passionate about and something that has helped keep the weight off. Always measure and/ or weigh every single portion no matter what.

As professional dieters, we think we know what equates to a tablespoon, two-thirds of a cup, or even four to six ounces of chicken breast. But the fact is we don't. And we may never get a grasp of this. If we really knew these measurements by heart, we probably wouldn't be in the position we're in. So please, trust me on this, measure everything you prepare for yourself from now until eternity.

I don't expect you to bring your measuring tools with you on vacation or when dining out or at a friend's house. Those are the times you can relax a little. But otherwise? Measure, measure, measure. Trust someone who took off and kept off over 250 pounds and who still measures his one cup of cereal *every* morning.

My other bit of advice is not to get caught up in the little diet myths we've been taught over the years. Somewhere along the way we bought the notion that avocado wasn't healthy, egg yolks were all wrong, peanuts were too filled with fat, and leaving the skin on the chicken makes babies cry.

Unless you have a specific food allergy or medical condition, it's okay to have the egg yolk (in moderation), avocado (healthy fat), or even nuts (super protein), and to enjoy the naturally occurring fat in chicken skin. Too often we focus on the little rules, which often leads to frustration, which then leads us to the nearest vat of ice cream.

Silly, silly stuff.

Breathe in. Breathe out. We are all works in progress. We're all learning as we go. And none of this is rocket science. It really can be this simple. The less we think about it, the less we agonize over it, the better. Stop over-thinking. Start doing. Today. This moment. Now.

No matter what plan you choose, I bet a few of my favorite recipes can be worked into it—before, during, or after your dieting phase.

Each of these recipes was a savior when it came to winning my own battle with the bulge. I needed my food to be healthy, easy-to-prepare, easy-to-freeze portions for future meals, and affordable. I hope you enjoy these recipes as much as I do. And yes, I still eat this stuff all the time.

GREGG'S CHUNKY TURKEY CHILI

This is a recipe I get asked about all the time. When I would have diet portions at work back during my days toiling away in the advertising department at Macy's, people would smell it and ask me for the recipe. I'll share the recipe with you, too.

Ingredients

5 tbsp. of extra virgin olive oil

3 white onions, peeled & chopped

2 7 oz. cans of diced green chilies (mild or hot—*your choice*)

3 tbsp. fresh garlic, chopped (can also used jarred, but without added oil)

4 tbsp. chili powder (more if you dare)

1 tbsp. ground cumin

1 tsp. ground cayenne pepper (more if you dare)

2+ lbs. low-fat ground turkey

1 6 lb., 6 oz. can (or several cans that equal the same) of ready cut diced tomatoes (in their own juice, no added sodium if available)

4 large bell peppers, chopped

Preparation

- In a large pot (the bigger the better), add the olive oil and chopped onions.
- Cover and cook over medium heat for several minutes (until the onions begin to soften).
- Next, add the garlic, chili powder and cumin.
- Mix it up and then add both cans (liquid and all) of the diced green chilies to the diced onion.
- Cook covered, over medium heat, for about 10 minutes.
- Next, add the ground turkey—making sure to mix all of the meat into the mixture while keeping the turkey from "clumping" together (work to break it up into loose pieces/bits).
- Continue to cook on medium heat for about 20 minutes, stirring occasionally (and de-clumping the turkey when necessary).
- Once the turkey is cooked through, add the canned tomatoes and chopped bell peppers.

- Mix thoroughly, then cover and cook on high heat until the contents reach a boil.
- As soon as you see that your mixture is boiling, reduce the heat to low and cook for about 20 minutes more so all the flavors mix together and blend to perfection.

Makes approximately 18 servings

Serving Suggestions

- Add a small green salad with carrot shavings and balsamic vinegar along with two to three multigrain crackers to create a complete meal.
- After preparing this big batch of chili, I divide it into portion sizes (usually two per storage container) and then, after the containers cool off, stick them in the freezer.
- After a day or so of thawing (in the fridge) you can zap it in the microwave for a quick, delicious dinner anytime during the week.
- You can store single size portions and take them to work for an easy and delicious microwavable lunch.

It should be noted that this turkey chili is so good you can even serve it to your friends and family members who aren't on a diet. Trust me; they'll never know they're eating something super healthy. I've even made a big batch of this recipe as a dip for parties and served it with multigrain chips along with sour cream and shredded cheese on the side.

GREGG'S BEST LUNCH SALAD EVER

Many dieters grow to resent having to rely on salads as their mainstay meal. But salads don't have to be boring. The key is adding texture, flavor, and even a little fat in a healthy form. The lunch salad recipe I'm sharing here is my go-to salad during the workweek. I have it daily, unless I have a lunch meeting that requires me to dine out, and never get tired of it. You can serve it to guests or other family members and they'll never suspect they're eating "diet food" given how tasty and delicious it is. What's more, it doubles as an excellent dinner salad. The only thing it's not good for? Breakfast. But then again . . . You never know.

Ingredients

For best flavor (and crunch appeal) use fresh ingredients whenever possible.

- 1 cup fresh arugula
- ½ cup fresh white corn kernels (cut from the cob just before serving)
- ½ cup cherry or grape tomatoes, sliced in half
- 1 piece of Gregg's Beer'd Chicken (prepared in advance. See page 268.)
- ¼ avocado, sliced lengthwise
- Balsamic vinegar
- Fresh ground pepper

Preparation

- Add ingredients to the plate, one at a time, building a small "pyramid" of sorts as you add the additional ingredients.
- After all ingredients are on the plate, add balsamic vinegar and fresh ground pepper to taste (those who aren't trying to take off excess weight can also add a drizzle of olive oil).
- Serve immediately.
- Makes 1 serving.
- Double, triple, quadruple, or whatever ingredients depending on number of guests.

GREGG'S BEER'D CHICKEN

I love making this chicken ahead of time and lots of it all at once as it lasts nearly a week and can be easily frozen and then just as easily reheated. It's just as delicious eaten hot as a main course as it is cold when cut into chunks for use in a lunch or dinner salad. You can also make this for friends. They'll be astounded at how moist and delicious this healthy entrée is.

I use chicken thighs instead of chicken breasts because I find the thighs offer a richer and moister flavor. Granted, there are a few more calories from fat in the thighs, but these aren't the kind of calories that get us into trouble. I also leave the skin on for some bonus flavor (both while cooking and while eating). If you're on a very strict plan, you can remove the skin, but do so after cooking so you still get the skin's benefits for the flavor.

Ingredients

6 to 12 large chicken thighs with skin

1 bottle of beer

Preparation

- Put chicken thighs into a large pot (bone down, skin side up).
- Pour a bottle of beer over the chicken thighs.
- Place a lid on the pot (preferably one that allows a minimal amount of airflow) and place the pot on the stovetop at the lowest heat.
- Cook on the lowest possible heat for about 2 to 4 hours (until chicken is slowly cooked through).
- While chicken is cooking, prepare a large broiling pan (I like lining the pan with parchment paper to make cleanup easier).
- Remove chicken from liquid and place on a broiling tray, skin-side-up (bone-side-down).
- Place tray under the broiler for approximately 8 minutes (on "high").
- After 8 minutes, remove the chicken from the broiler. Allow chicken to sit for a few minutes. Then it's ready to serve (or store in fridge for future use).

Makes 6 to 12 servings (depending on the number and size of the thighs)

For me, a common evening meal will include one to two pieces of Beer'd Chicken (sprinkled with a splash of balsamic vinegar, then covered and warmed up in the oven on low heat for approximately twenty minutes if coming from the fridge), along with steamed green beans (sprinkled with granulated garlic, fresh ground pepper, and a few splashes of balsamic vinegar), and a ½-cup of cherry or grape tomatoes (each sliced in half).

Another option is to serve the chicken with my "Fresh Veggie Side Salad" recipe for a winning and complete meal. Your taste buds will thank me for it. If you'd like the recipe for the side salad, see page 270.

GREGG'S FRESH VEGGIE SIDE SALAD

This side salad is tasty, hearty, and a real crowd pleaser. What's more, it's so healthy you don't have to avoid it when on a diet or another type of healthy eating program. But at the same time, because it tastes so good, you don't have to "doctor it up" for guests who might not be watching their weight.

Ingredients

4   ears of corn

1   avocado (large, ripe, but firm—not mushy)

2   pints cherry or grape tomatoes

Olive oil

Balsamic vinegar

Fresh ground pepper to taste

Preparation

- Remove the kernels from corn cob with sharp knife and place freshly cut kernels in bowl.
- Rinse cherry or grape tomatoes, cut into halves, add all to bowl with the corn kernels.
- Peel avocado, cut into small chunks, add to bowl with corn and tomatoes.
- Add 4 tablespoons of olive oil, 2 tablespoons of balsamic vinegar, pepper to taste.
- Toss together and serve immediately.

Makes 6 servings

This also makes a great dish to bring to any party. I promise it will be a big hit. Double the recipe and make it shortly before you leave. Do not add olive oil, balsamic vinegar, or pepper until just before serving.

STEAK À LA GREGG

Looking to cook up some mouth-watering, diet-friendly steaks that are as healthy as they are delicious (assuming eating red meat in moderation is part of your healthy eating plan)? Well, look no further because I'm going to share my tried-and-true recipe for creating delicious steaks that are sure to please any dieter as well as any dinner guest.

I usually fix these steaks on Sunday nights as a special weekend treat. The best part is that when having guests over I don't have to do anything different to "dress up" their steaks. Easy. Fast. Delicious. Just a broiler and a few spices needed. And no outdoor grill is necessary, though you could certainly use a grill if you have one handy.

First things first: Look for steaks that are red, juicy, and fresh. Always check the expiration date and never purchase steaks that are about to "expire," look dull in color, or ones that are starting to gray. The steaks should have fat veins running through the meat as well as some fat around the edges. There isn't any additional butter or oil with this recipe, so the fat in the steak helps with the flavor while making the steaks virtually self-basting while broiling and extremely juicy and tender for eating.

Not to worry, this naturally occurring fat won't harm your healthy eating plan when enjoyed in moderation. Remember, it's all about balance.

I usually prefer big, thick rib eye steaks. And the cuts of meat I use are large. As you'll read later, each of the steaks I buy make for more than one serving, which makes for convenient leftover meals during the week.

Ingredients

2–4 rib eye steaks (depending on number of guests;
you can always just prepare 1 steak, too)
Granulated garlic
Fresh ground pepper

Preparation

- Preheat broiler to highest setting.
- Ready a shallow, nonstick, broiler-safe baking pan (not a baking sheet).

- Place steaks in pan.
- Cover each steak generously with granulated garlic and fresh ground pepper.
- Broil for 10–17 minutes, depending on thickness of meat.
- Remove pan from broiler, turn steaks over, re-sprinkle with garlic and pepper (be mindful of the sometimes bubbling liquefied fat).
- Broil for 5–7 minutes more (depending on desired cooking temperature).
- Remove from broiler (again, taking care with the sometimes bubbling liquefied fat).
- Carefully remove steak from broiling pan, place on doubled paper towel (on plate).
- Put another doubled-paper towel on other side, then "press" steak (which is now between the paper towels) with spatula (this soaks up most of the "fat juice" from the steak, but still leaves it moist with a little bit of running liquid).
- Remove paper towels, turn steak over (so the first side cooked faces up for "best presentation" purposes).
- Add side salad (see page 270).
- Serve immediately.

Makes 2 to 4 servings (plus leftovers)

Additional Tip

As always, you want to keep portion control in mind. I usually eat about half of my steak and save the rest for an easy midweek meal, chopping up the remaining portion in a salad or simply warming it up and serving it with steamed vegetables and freshly sliced cherry or grape tomatoes. If you think you might overdo it (eat too much), then cut your steak portion in half before serving.

Also, because I know I will be reheating the saved portion of the steak later in the week, I usually undercook my steak a little, and avoid eating the less cooked part of it (the more rare part near the center) during the first serving.

GREGG'S SUMMER FRUIT SALAD

This fresh summer salad is a healthy and delicious treat you can easily toss together for special events. Bring it to every social occasion or picnic so you'll have something you can enjoy without worry. This way you can stay on your plan and no one will worry that you're "not eating at the party."

Salad Ingredients

    6   cups of fresh, chopped, seedless watermelon
    2   cups of fresh blueberries
    2   cups of fresh, sliced strawberries
    2   cups of green, seedless grapes (each sliced in half)
    1   cup of fresh blackberries

Dressing Ingredients

    ½   cup fresh, pure orange juice
    1   tbsp. fresh or organic lemon juice
    1   tsp. ground ginger

Preparation

- Chop and mix all ingredients as close to serving time as possible (that way the fruit will stay crisp).
- Store in freezer for half hour before serving.
- Just before putting it out for guests (or for yourself), toss dressing and mix with fruit, then serve. You can also serve without dressing depending on how sweet and ripe the fruit is.

Makes 8 servings

Be sure to pay attention to serving size if you're on any kind of diet plan.

GREGG'S GUILT-FREE SWORDFISH

Next time someone suggests you "Go fish," do just that with this surprisingly easy swordfish recipe that can entice even those who don't list seafood as a favorite main dish.

Ingredients

Swordfish steak

Granulated garlic (not garlic salt)

Balsamic vinegar

Fresh ground pepper

Preparation

- Preheat broiler.
- Place swordfish on nonstick surface, sprinkle lightly with granulated garlic and fresh ground pepper, add several drops of balsamic vinegar.
- Broil on high for 6 to 7 minutes, then turn over fish, sprinkle on a few more droplets of balsamic vinegar and broil for approximately 5 to 6 more minutes (depending on the thickness of the cut).
- Use a spatula to move fish to plate. It will be moist and delicious without any need for added oil, butter, or salt.
- Try serving it with fresh cherry or grape tomatoes (sliced into halves, sprinkled with fresh ground pepper).
- Add a slice or two of lemon as a garnish.

Makes 1 serving

SOME FINAL THOUGHTS ON EATING "RIGHT"

Be careful of "diet foods" marketed directly toward those of us who are trying to be healthy. Just because it has a green package—the food industry's "signal" that it's a "healthier" choice—doesn't necessarily mean it's healthy for you. The fresher, more natural, and more pure your food is, the easier your body can digest it and the more effective your metabolism will be.

The incredible amounts of salt, preservatives, and artificial ingredients used to "enhance" certain packaged foods have the potential to be poison to your system. Your body doesn't necessarily know how to process these additives. You'll discover that you feel better and look better if you eat food that is fresh and pure, without any artificial ingredients or additives.

This new look won't be limited to just your body size. Your skin will glow. Your hair will shine. Your overall feeling of wellness will improve vastly.

Of course there's more to getting rid of excess weight than nutrition and portion control. Like it or not, we have to start moving. And yes, that means exercise. A lot of us lifetime dieters have never incorporated daily or weekly exercise into our lives. At the risk of overusing a phrase—if I can do it, anyone can do it. (And that means *you, too!*)

2. MOVE MORE

I'll say it again: An essential part of your success is exercise. It's not an *optional* part of getting healthy. It's a must! By moving your body, you're kick-starting your metabolism, burning fat, and building muscle.

What's more, you're going to be improving your inner health—heart, organs, muscles, joints—you name it. There's no excuse not to exercise, no matter what your fitness level. It's a good idea to check in with your medical professional to discuss the best kind of exercise for you to start out with if you're just beginning a workout regimen. Trust me, this step is worth it, and it might even be able to take place via telephone. Remember, we're talking about your overall health here, so a little homework will absolutely be worth the effort.

The key is being smart about exercise. This means doing what's reasonable for your current body type and your current state of health. You don't want to hurt yourself or end up experiencing pain or discomfort.

Exercising should be fun. Not only will it increase your energy, it will cause endorphins to surge through your body, which can dramatically improve your mood. Endorphins are nature's antidepressant.

Exercise can also help balance out your metabolism. If you're anything like me, you've started and stopped lots of different diets over and over. This can really confuse your natural metabolism and make your whole "system" slow down. Exercise helps kick this system back into gear. In fact, it helps your body function better on almost every level.

And the best part? Exercise does as much for your outward appearance as it does for your internal health. There's nothing wrong with letting your vanity fuel your efforts. It's what kept me motivated long enough to start my journey to a healthier self. Exercise is going to help uncover your fiercest self sooner rather than later.

When you're exercising in conjunction with your eating plan, you're doubling your efforts and speeding up your results. If you have to, start slow (and safe). But definitely *start* . . . today!

POSTURE IS EVERYTHING

Make sure you don't live life in a slump, whether you're working at your desk, cooking in the kitchen, running an errand, or exercising. Stand up tall, pull your shoulders back, suck in your stomach, and keep your head held high (imagine carrying a stack of books on the top of your head).

Making sure you keep proper posture during exercise and all other tasks of daily living will not only increase your exercise's effectiveness, it will also improve your overall health and appearance.

WALK THE WALK

The best exercise for every fitness level is also the easiest to do—walking. The key is to walk with proper posture and to pump your arms back and forth while taking steps. Those at lower fitness levels can pace themselves and start out slowly. Even just ten minutes, four days a week will be beneficial. Then add more time to those ten-minute sessions each week.

Make sure you always suck in your stomach while you walk. You want to work those muscles constantly. If you walk with proper posture and suck in your stomach the whole time, you will not only burn calories, but also work your abdominal muscles. And don't forget to pump those arms.

Remember, you're not out taking a casual stroll. You're working your body and working it hard. Try and work up to a pace that will cause you to break a sweat. Use the time for what it's meant for: Transforming your body.

Soon, you can be power walking forty-five to sixty minutes each time you work out, as well as making a huge difference in your weight loss efforts. The best part is that you don't need a treadmill or even a gym membership to take advantage of walking (though either can make for a great investment in yourself).

You can walk around your neighborhood and simply keep moving in place when you reach a traffic light and have to wait to cross the street. You can also drive to a local park or, better yet, a hiking trail that offers hills, which can be great for your legs and gluteal muscles. If the weather's rainy or cold, get yourself to the nearest mall. Senior citizens have been doing mall walks for years, and it's dramatically improved their health. You can do the same thing no matter what age you are. Most malls open earlier to accommodate walkers. Call the management office of your local indoor shopping centers to find out if they offer such hours. If outdoors, make sure you're dressed properly for the weather. And no matter where you're walking, make sure you're outfitted in a pair of comfortable and supportive walking shoes or sneakers.

For those of you who do happen to belong to a gym or own a treadmill, treadmills can be great "partners" for your walking workout. Try setting the incline higher than level and walk with speed up a simulated hill. Try to not hold on to the machine. You will see people at the gym reading magazines, holding on, or walking and talking. I believe this hampers the health benefits of walking on a treadmill.

You are there to work out. Pump your arms, suck in your stomach, breathe properly, and work your body. You're not there to socialize or show someone your new sneakers. You're there to transform your body. Soon you'll be feeling all the physical and mental benefits that exercise delivers. And then there's going to be no stopping you from reaching your goals.

WORKOUT PARTNERS

Working out with a buddy is a fun and helpful thing to do. You can both motivate one another. But if your friend isn't able to make your workout date, still get out there on your own. There are no excuses for not moving and exercising. Sometimes the best workout partner comes in the form of an iPod or the MP3 player on your smart phone. Put your favorite music on there and create a playlist of songs that inspire you to move.

MUSCLE TRAINING

It's important to incorporate resistance training (weightlifting, etc.) into your workouts. By adding resistance training to your routine, you'll build up muscle mass. This will result not just in looking better and feeling better, but also in increasing your body's ability to burn more calories throughout the day.

Muscle mass requires more internal fuel to maintain than non-muscle mass, meaning that people with defined muscles burn more calories even when they're sleeping. There are other great reasons to have muscle mass in your body, too. It makes you stronger, healthier, and more confident. You can purchase your own hand weights from sports supply stores or join a gym when you're ready to do so or when you can afford to join. Yes, a gym membership costs money, but think of the long-term health benefits that you will gain.

THE FOUNTAIN OF YOUTH

One of the most powerful additions I've made to my own exercise program is the practice of yoga. I was resistant to it at first. It was challenging for me to quiet my mind and to go through the paces with the rest of the class. But soon I learned to love yoga for its mind-transforming benefits as well as its rewards for my body and internal organs.

I found nothing transformed my formerly fat body into a leaner, sexier, and more defined one like yoga did. Even after years of other forms of exercise, I found yoga's benefits could be seen almost immediately. Classes for every level are available at gyms, community centers, and even on DVDs. Try renting a couple different DVDs until you find one that works for you, then buy that one.

When you look around at those who attend yoga classes, you'll be amazed at the range of ages of the students. I'm always impressed and inspired by people in their sixties and seventies who are able to do poses more elegantly and athletically than I can. They look amazing. Their glowing skin, vibrant hair, and healthy body shapes offer pure inspiration. I suggest adding yoga to every exercise program. It has the potential to transform your life.

THE TWO MOST IMPORTANT WORDS ABOUT WORKING OUT:
NO EXCUSES!

When I was taking off more than 250 pounds, I was working full-time in New York City while living in New Jersey. I had a lengthy commute each way, and was expected to be at the office for about ten hours a day. This meant I was away from home for almost thirteen hours, yet I still found time to work out.

I'm not bragging. I'm just letting you know there are no excuses for not working out. I don't care how busy you are. If you're *really committed* to this change, you're going to find time. It might be when the kids are finally asleep. It might be at the crack of dawn, or even before the crack of dawn.

I get up at 4:30 every morning to exercise. When you're committed, you make time. You find time. You do what you have to do. And you should be committed. After all, we're talking about an amazing change for your body, your health, and your life.

No excuses! Exercise three to four times a week. It's essential.

3. DRINK PLENTY OF WATER

A lot of people are surprised when I list drinking lots of water as one of the necessary steps to getting rid of the excess weight. Take it from someone who used to quench his thirst with lots of soda—first the sugar-filled kind and then the diet kind. Frankly, I'm not sure which was worse for me. I found soda to be very addictive, so getting "off" of it was difficult.

Drinking enough water to help with my weight loss and ensure I was properly hydrated was equally difficult. I was never one to sip on water. Given this, I learned to just go to the kitchen—at home, at work, at a friend's house—and gulp down a glass of water, usually at room temperature, whenever I would think of it. I would manually keep track of how many glasses I was drinking a day until I hit the magic number, which for me was—and still is—around ten glasses a day.

Starting your own "water habit" may not be easy, but trust me when I say it's essential. If you don't believe me, ask your doctor about how important drinking water is or, at the very least, look it up online.

Yes, you will likely be in the bathroom a little more than you're used to, but staying hydrated is worth it. As you diet and lose weight, you want to flush out your fat cells and clean out your system. Water is the way to do this effectively and safely. Plus, it helps you stay full. Additionally, water will help with occasional headaches that can occur when first starting a healthier eating regimen.

If you're not used to drinking water, get used to it. You want to be fit and healthy, right? Then start gulping the water. Your body will thank you for it.

I begin every single day with an eight-ounce glass of filtered room temperature water with fresh or organic lemon juice squeezed into it. This wakes up my metabolism and also offers a great way to instantly rehydrate after a good night's sleep.

DON'T CONFUSE HUNGER FOR THIRST

Often times, when it *feels* like you're hungry, you're actually thirsty. Again, it's important for people who are shedding weight to drink plenty of water, not just to stay hydrated but to flush toxins from the body and aid in flushing fat cells.

It's important you drink water throughout the day, including before and after working out. Those of you who choose to drink coffee or green tea will need a little more water to balance out the caffeine that's in your system, which can sometimes act as a diuretic.

HOW MUCH WATER TO DRINK

Need to know how much water is enough for you? The average person should drink eight to ten eight-ounce glasses of water a day. That equals about two-and-a-half quarts of water. Medical professionals often recommend that people who want to lose weight should drink an added glass of water for every twenty-five pounds of excess weight they're currently carrying on their body. The amount of water consumed should also be increased when exercising or when the weather is very warm.

Remember, water doesn't have to be boring. Try adding a little organic or fresh squeezed lemon juice to filtered water for more flavor. You can also drink sparkling water. Just make sure it has no additives (some seltzers contain sodium).

And again, when you're drinking enough water, you're going to be using the restroom frequently. This is actually very healthy. Just make sure you plan your water drinking for times when you'll be near an easy-to-access bathroom.

SPA WATER RECIPE

It's easy to make something I call Spa Water, which has become a favorite of guests, no matter the social occasion. Take a pitcher of filtered water, add ten fresh cucumber slices. Next, cut a washed lemon (or even an orange, your choice) into wedges and squeeze the juice into the pitcher, then add the squeezed lemon wedge. Cover the pitcher and let it sit in the fridge for about twenty-four hours. The resulting water will be crisp, cool, and flavorful—a real pick-me-up and something of a treat. Serve over ice with a fresh-cut lemon wedge on the glass as a garnish.

A Few More Reasons to Drink Lots of Water

1. Water can help us feel more satiated (often when we think we're hungry, we're just dehydrated).
2. Water has the potential to help our bodies metabolize fat more efficiently.
3. Water can enhance muscle tone.
4. Water helps keep skin looking fresh and can give it a natural "glow."
5. Water is essential for eliminating waste as well as combating bloating.

4. GET PLENTY OF SLEEP

Medical professionals universally proclaim that getting enough sleep is essential to our overall health. You may have seen news stories and recent studies connecting proper amounts of sleep with maintaining a healthy weight. So why wouldn't it be necessary for our bodies when we're trying to lose excess weight and get healthier in general?

Pay attention to how you feel after eating certain kinds of foods, drinking certain kinds of drinks, and doing certain kinds of workouts. It's all about getting in touch with how we feel—both mentally and physically. And the less chemical and artificial substances we consume, the easier it will be to sleep, and the more we will crave sleep because we just might be getting real rest for the first time in a long time.

I know that during my years of being morbidly obese, I didn't sleep well, often waking up due to indigestion, night sweats, or mental stress. The healthier I became, the better I was able to sleep and the more rested and capable of accomplishing anything I felt in the morning.

Make sure you schedule enough time for enough sleep—seven to eight hours at least. Your body will go through amazing changes on your healthy eating plan, and it will need rest to achieve the desired results. I know we all lead busy lives and it's easy to "steal time" from bedtime. But you're only hurting yourself when you do this. Think of a good night's sleep as a way to refuel your body in order to be able to handle whatever comes your way. Remember, losing the excess weight won't mean a thing in the long run if you're not feeling as good as you're looking. So be kind to your body, mind, and soul. Getting enough sleep is essential to your success.

LAST, BUT NOT LEAST

Go easy on yourself. Be gentle with yourself. Remember that Rome wasn't built in a day. Think of the changes you're initiating as more of a *life plan* than a *diet plan*. Take things step-by-step and try not to think of being "on" or "off" ("cheating" or "not cheating"). Think instead of turning the page and starting a new chapter. A chapter in which you can enjoy everything life has to offer—in moderation.

Moderation has become my key word for just about everything (even, sadly, my wacky sense of humor). Too much of anything can equate to overdoing it. But just enough? That can often be just right.

No matter what odds you're facing, you do have what it takes. And given that, I encourage you to chronicle your journey.

As I mentioned earlier, while on my own weight loss journey, I bought a large, blank scrapbook, which can easily be found in bookstores and art supply stores. I then used this Me Book as a success scrapbook, cutting out words I found inspiring, articles about health and fitness, pictures from catalogs featuring "average sized clothes" that I wanted to wear and so on, and then pasting them onto the pages of my Me Book. I even put my "before" picture into this book and kept track of my weekly weight loss.

My scrapbook became a real source of inspiration for me throughout my weight loss adventure. After all, I was on a journey. Chronicling that journey was not only therapeutic but also extremely inspirational. I suggest you do the same. It is something you create yourself that is all about you and your reasons for taking off the unwanted pounds. Think of it as a vision board you can add to, look at, and take with you wherever you go. I used to pick my scrapbook up all the time when I was tempted to stray from my eating plan. And today? It serves as an amazing testament to what I went through, not only taking off the weight, but keeping it off. These days, an inspiration collection like this could also be created on Pinterest.

Get a book right away, or start a board on Pinterest. Then keep your eye out for anything you find inspiring—from magazines, catalogs, letters from friends, Internet printouts, etc. There are no rules. This is your book. Your inspiration. And when you reach your goal, you'll have a testament to not only your journey, but also your success.

Hear that applause in the distance? That's me, clapping for you. It doesn't matter how many times you've tried to lose weight (or whatever) before. It doesn't matter that you've sometimes crashed and burned. It doesn't matter that you've made decisions in the past that you'd make differently now.

Everything in your life, even the seemingly tragic moments, has made you who you are today. And you have the capability to be everything you want to be. In this very moment you are there. Start living like that and you'll see that everything else can fall into place. You might even be surprised at how quickly it happens.

Just like me, everyone has the power to be weightless. And that, my friend, definitely includes *you*.